Studying
HEALTH&
DISEASE

prepared by the
Open University's U205 Course Team

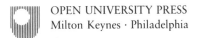
OPEN UNIVERSITY PRESS
Milton Keynes · Philadelphia

The U205 Course Team

U205 is a course whose writing and production has been the joint effort of many hands, a 'core course team', and colleagues who have written on specific aspects of the course but have not been involved throughout; together with editors, designers, and the BBC team.

Core Course Team

The following people have written or commented extensively on the whole course, been involved in all phases of its production and accept collective responsibility for its overall academic and teaching content.

Steven Rose (neurobiologist; course team chair; academic editor; Book VI coordinator)

Nick Black (community physician; Book IV coordinator)

Basiro Davey (immunologist; course manager; Book V coordinator)

Alastair Gray (health economist; Book III coordinator)

Kevin McConway (statistician; Book I coordinator)

Jennie Popay (social policy analyst; Book VIII coordinator)

Jacqueline Stewart (managing editor)

Phil Strong (medical sociologist; academic editor; Book II coordinator)

Other authors

The following authors have contributed to the overall development of the course and have taken responsibility for writing specific sections of it.

Lynda Birke (ethologist; author, Book V)

Eric Bowers (parasitologist; staff tutor)

David Boswell (sociologist; author, Book II; Book VII coordinator)

Eva Chapman (psychotherapist; author, Book V)

Andrew Learmonth (geographer; course team chair 1983; author, Book III)

Rosemary Lennard (medical practitioner; author, Books IV and V)

Jim Moore (historian of science; author, Book II)

Sean Murphy (neurobiologist; author, Book VI)

Rob Ransom (developmental biologist; author, Book IV)

George Watts (historian; author, Book II)

The following people have assisted with particular aspects or parts of the course.

Sylvia Bentley (course secretary)

Steve Best (illustrator)

Sheila Constantinou (BBC production assistant)

Ann Hall (indexer)

Rachel Hardman (designer)

Mark Kesby (illustrator)

Liz Lane (editor)

Vic Lockwood (BBC producer)

Laurie Melton (librarian)

Sue Walker (editor)

Peter Wright (editor)

External consultant

Sheila M. Gore (medical statistician) Medical Research Council Biostatistics Unit, Cambridge.

External Assessors

Course Assessor

Alwyn Smith President, Faculty of Community Medicine of the Royal Colleges of Physicians; Professor of Epidemiology and Social Oncology, University of Manchester.

Book I Assessor

Klim McPherson Lecturer in Medical Statistics, Department of Community Medicine and General Practice, University of Oxford.

Acknowledgements

The course team wishes to thank the following for their advice and contributions:

Sheila Adam (community physician) North West Thames Regional Health Authority.

John Ashton (community physician) Department of Community Health, University of Liverpool.

Graham Burchell (philosopher) Westminster College of Education.

Angela Coulter (sociologist) Department of Community Medicine and General Practice, University of Oxford.

Barbara Harrison (sociologist) Department of Sociology, Polytechnic of South Bank.

Ann McPherson (general practitioner) Oxford.

Ann Murcott (sociologist) Department of Sociology, University of Cardiff; Department of Psychological Medicine; Welsh National School of Medicine.

Andrew Neil (community physician) Department of Community Medicine and General Practice, University of Oxford.

Hilary Rose (sociologist) Department of Applied Social Studies, University of Bradford.

Open University Press, Celtic Court, 22 Ballmoor, Buckingham, MK18 1XW.

First published 1985. Reprinted 1986, 1990. Copyright © The Open University.

Designed by the Graphic Design Group of the Open University.

Typeset by the Pindar Group of Companies, Scarborough, North Yorkshire. Printed by St Edmundsbury Press Ltd, Bury St Edmunds, Suffolk.

ISBN 0 335 15050 0

This book forms part of the Open University Press 'Health and Disease' series. The complete list of books in the series is printed on the back cover.

Further information on Open University courses may be obtained from the Admissions Office, The Open University, P.O. Box 48, Walton Hall, Milton Keynes, MK7 6AB.

About this book

A note for t_____
*Studying Hea*_____
on the subjec_____
so that it can_____ ...ke any other textbook,
or studied as_____ ...0205 *Health and Disease*, a second
level course for Open University students. As well as the
eight textbooks and a Course Reader, *Health and Disease:
A Reader,** the course consists of eleven TV programmes
and five audiocassettes plus various supplementary
materials.

Open University students will receive an *Introduction
and Guide* to the course, which sets out a study plan for the
year's work. This is supplemented where appropriate in the
text by more detailed directions for OU students; these
study comments at the beginning of chapters are boxed for
ease of reference. Also, in the text you will find instructions
to refer to the Course Reader. It is quite possible to follow
the argument without reading the articles referred to,
although your understanding will be enriched if you do so.
Major learning objectives are listed at the end of each
chapter along with questions that allow students to assess
how well they are achieving those objectives. The index
includes key words (in bold type) which can be looked up
easily as an aid to revision as the course proceeds. There is
also a further reading list for those who wish to pursue
certain aspects of study beyond the limits of this book.

A guide for OU students

In *Studying Health and Disease* we set out a variety of
approaches to study health and disease: clinical and
biological, epidemiological and social, quantitative and
qualitative. We discuss methodology, that is how we

* Black, Nick *et al.* (1984) *Health and Disease: A Reader*, Open
University Press.

...acts and ...test hypotheses in the social and
...logical sciences. Later books of the course will give an
overall description of the 'facts' about health and disease as
seen by biologists, or by social scientists; here we are mainly
concerned with the methods they use to arrive at these
'facts'.

Book I falls roughly into three main parts preceded by
an introduction. Chapters 2 and 3 are concerned with the
clinical method and with disease as a biological
phenomenon. In Chapters 4–6 questions about the
distribution of health and disease are addressed through
epidemiology and statistics. The third main subject is the
techniques used in looking at the social context of health
and disease (Chapters 7–10). Finally, Chapters 11 and 12
provide links between the three main areas of discussion.

We have planned for you to work through Chapters 1–3
and then to turn to Book II, *Medical Knowledge: Doubt
and Certainty*, and complete that before coming back to
study Chapters 4–12 of this book. Chapters 1–3 describe
the traditional approaches to health and disease, focused
around individuals. Though these techniques are extremely
powerful, they do not tell the whole story. Book II
demonstrates that we cannot understand sickness wholely
by focusing on the biology of the individual but need a fully
biosocial approach. Having established this, we ask you to
return to methods of studying groups and societies in
Chapters 4–12 of this book.

The time allowed for studying Books I and II is 6 weeks
or 60 hours. Chapters 1–3 should take approximately half
a week and Chapters 4–12 around two and a half weeks.
The following table gives a more detailed breakdown to
help you to pace your study. You need not follow it
slavishly but do not allow yourself to fall behind. If you find
a section of the work difficult, do what you can at this stage,
and return to rework the material at the end of your study
of the two books.

Study time for Book I (total 30 hours)

Chapter	Time/hours	Course Reader	Time/hours	TV and audiocassettes	Time/hours
1	$\frac{1}{4}$ ⎫				
2	$1\frac{3}{4}$ ⎬ $4\frac{1}{2}$			none associated with Book I	
3	$2\frac{1}{2}$ ⎭				

NOW STUDY BOOK II = 30 hours (3 weeks); see 'About this book' for Book II.

Chapter	Time/hours	Course Reader	Time/hours	TV and audiocassettes	Time/hours
4	$4\frac{1}{2}$ ⎫				
5	$4\frac{1}{2}$ ⎬ 13				
6	4 ⎭	Smithells *et al.* (1980) Laurence *et al.* (1981)	1		
7	1 ⎫				
8	1 ⎬ $4\frac{3}{4}$				
9	$1\frac{1}{2}$	van den Berg (1981)	$\frac{1}{2}$		
10	$1\frac{1}{4}$ ⎭				
11	3 ⎫ $3\frac{1}{4}$				
12	$\frac{1}{4}$ ⎭				

Assessment There is a TMA (tutor-marked assignment) associated with this book; three hours have been allowed for its completion.

Final note You will find an electronic calculator (a very simple one will do) useful for Chapters 4 and 5.

Contents

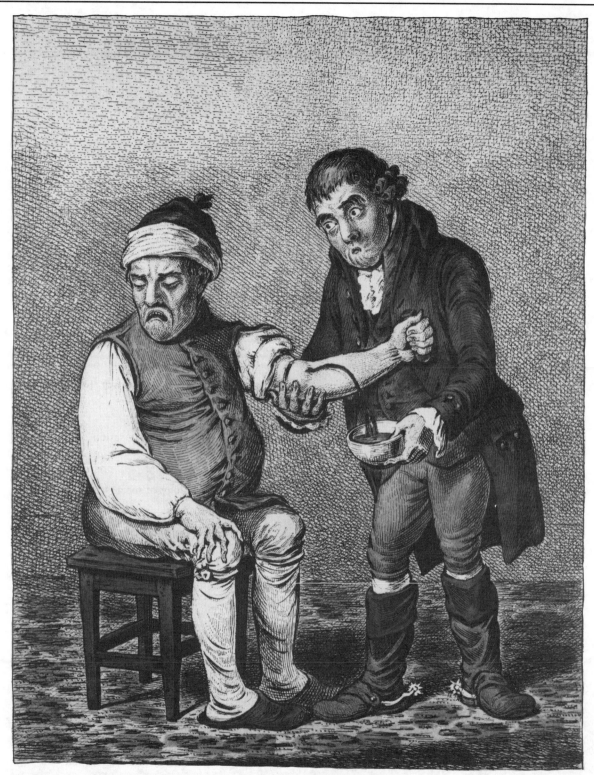

Blood-letting, one of the techniques frequently used in Britain before the rise of scientific medicine.

1
Introduction

This book is about discovering how to explain health and disease and about understanding the relationships between different types of explanation. Time and time again in your own experience, you will have come across what seem to be conflicting and mutually exclusive interpretations of these phenomena. How can such apparently conflicting explanations for disease, from the common cold to schizophrenia, be reconciled?

☐ Think back to the last time you had a cold. Why did you have a cold? What caused it? Write down as many different ways as you can think of to complete the sentence: 'I had a cold because ...'

■ Here are some examples of the kind of answers people might give.

'I had a cold because I got my feet wet.'

'I had a cold because I was run down, because my firm had been making me work too hard.'

'I had a cold because I hadn't been eating properly.'

'I had a cold because I went to visit my brother who had a cold and caught it from him.'

'I had a cold because a virus got into my nose and throat.'

'I had a cold because cells in my nasal passages were malfunctioning.'

'I had a cold because there was a lot of it going round at the time in our town.'

Of course, there are many more possible answers.

Can all these answers be 'true', or is only one of them the 'real' explanation? How can we distinguish true from false explanations: 'I had a cold because a virus infected me' from 'I had a cold because an ill-wisher put a spell on me'? And if we can distinguish different types of causes of a cold, how could we distinguish between the effectiveness of possible *treatments*? 'When I caught cold I went on working as if nothing had happened and took a whole week to recover.' 'I went to bed with a hot-water bottle and drank half a bottle of whisky a day and recovered within seven days.' Some people swear by vitamin C, others avoid draughts and damp.

Let us look at the explanations more closely and try to sort them into categories. In some explanations the fact that the person has a cold is seen in terms of what is happening in the present to certain parts of the person — a malfunction of cells in the nasal passages — or what is happening to the individual — 'I had a cold because I was run down' — or what is happening to a group of people in which the individual is included — 'a lot of it going around at the time in our town'. Each of these explanations attempts to describe what is happening to a person at a different level: the level of component parts of the person, or of the individual, or of groups of people of which the person concerned is a member.

But more often the cold is viewed as a consequence of something that happened in the *past*, for example getting wet feet, not eating properly, the visit to a sick brother or becoming run down because of overwork. Getting wet feet and not eating well involve directly only the individual concerned. The former is a purely physical event but the latter is perhaps more to do with the individual's lifestyle and psychological makeup. The other two explanations involve interaction with other people, either in biological terms (visiting another human who is infected) or in social terms (the slave-driving firm). How do all these explanations relate to each other? Although they are so different at first glance, they do not necessarily contradict each other. It might be that all are valid. Part of the task of this book is to describe ways in which they may indeed be valid.

So health and disease can be discussed and explained at different levels: we can focus on the past or the present, on individuals, or component parts of individuals or groups of individuals ranging right up to societies and nations. All of these discussions can contribute to people's understanding of their own health and ill-health, to solving individual problems and to solving social problems.

A major approach to sorting the explanations is to distinguish between those that locate the cause of the cold inside the individual, as a malfunctioning of their biology, and those that seek explanations in the wider social framework. The former type of explanation is the most familiar *medical* approach. It is committed to the concept of individual diseases, which medicine defines as collections of signs and symptoms. Once medicine has done this defining, it is the task of the biological sciences to locate the causes of these disease entities in specific phenomena such as genetic abnormality, an infective microorganism, or whatever.

The alternative type of explanation requires investigation by the social sciences and through the study of epidemiology. This type of explanation seeks an answer to why diseases such as colds are more prevalent in particular parts of the country or in particular social classes. Are women more prone to colds than men? And what about people in particular jobs? Answering such questions involves the measurement of the number of people affected by particular diseases at particular times and in particular places and an attempt to discuss what the people who are affected (or unaffected) have in common. This involves the study of health statistics.

In this book, the first type of explanation, the medical and biological, forms the theme of Chapters 2 and 3. The second type of approach, of epidemiology and the social sciences, is discussed in Chapters 4–10. In Chapters 11 and 12, we try to put the two types of explanation together again in a model that endeavours to synthesise the themes of biology, of the social order and of a crucial third dimension, personal life history.

But before it is possible to begin to adjudicate between different explanations, whether of a cold or of any other disease, it is necessary to have methods of observation and of measurement. The types of explanation offered in this book have one thing in common: they all involve observing things happening. Yet observation does not itself provide explanations. We shall discuss methods of doing the observing, methods of producing an explanation from what is observed, the problems of deciding whether an explanation is true or false, and the problems of relating one type of explanation to another. The theme of methods of observation, of determining the answers to such questions, is taken up in Chapters 4–10. There we approach issues of how frequent certain diseases are in the population, of how much ill-health is or is not reported to doctors, of simple quantitative questions such as how many days are lost from work for colds or anything else each year, and of qualitative questions such as how bad was the cold, how ill did it make a person feel? For only on the basis of observation and measurement can one begin to distinguish true explanations from false. Also these techniques are essential in the evaluation of treatments of diseases.

You might question why we have chosen to start our study of health and disease this way, rather than beginning with 'the facts' about health and disease in our world. We have done this because we think that to understand an observation, it is necessary to understand something about how the observation was made and about why the observer chose to make that particular observation rather than another. We certainly do not intend that you should become a competent *user* of all the methods we describe in this book — reading Chapter 2 will not qualify you to practise as a doctor, for example! Instead, our aim is that you should become *aware* of the methods of enquiry used in studying health and disease, and in particular of their strengths and limitations. The problems and examples discussed in this book are there because we think they provide clear illustrations of the methods discussed, and not because they are necessarily the most important problems in their particular field. Other books of the course will provide an overview of health and disease as seen by biologists and by social scientists. That overview will allow you to test out in practice how convincing — or otherwise — you find the attempt at 'synthesising' the reductionist, holistic and historical explanations of health and disease that we make in later chapters of this book.

In discussing the various types of explanation of disease we have chosen as a unifying illustration the causes and treatments of a particular disease, diabetes. But what *is* diabetes; is it a single disease? And what is disease anyway? Let us begin at what is for most of us in the UK today, the start of our quest for answers to questions of health and disease, the doctor's consulting room . . . .

2
The clinical method

Diabetes mellitus is used in this chapter (and throughout the book) purely for illustrative purposes; you are not expected to learn the specific features of this condition.

Robert Lawson, a fifty-seven year old plumber who had previously enjoyed good health, went to see his doctor one evening because he had recently been suffering from pains in his legs. His doctor questioned him about the nature, severity and frequency of these pains, about whether he had any other problems with his health and about how things in general were going at work and at home. Mr Lawson reported that he had 'not been feeling himself' recently and in addition had been troubled by the minor inconvenience of having to get up at night to pass urine. The doctor examined Mr Lawson's legs, feeling for lumps, areas of tenderness and arterial pulses. She also checked to see: if there was any loss of sensation in his legs (testing first with a pin, and then with a vibrating tuning-fork); whether there was any painful restriction of leg movement; and whether the knee and ankle reflexes were normal. Finally, using an ophthalmoscope, she examined Mr Lawson's eyes.

The doctor then explained that she would like to test a specimen of Mr Lawson's urine. She did this by dipping a stick coated with a mixture of chemicals into the urine sample. (The chemicals change colour depending on the amount of sugar present in the sample.) This test revealed that there was sugar in Mr Lawson's urine (not usually present). In the light of this, the doctor asked him if he could come to see her again in the morning for a blood test before he had anything to eat. The consultation ended with the doctor explaining that the leg pains may be due to diabetes and that the following day's test would show whether or not this is correct.

Diabetes mellitus (usually just referred to as diabetes) is a condition in which the control of the use of sugar (glucose) in the body is disordered in such a way that sugar appears in high levels in the blood and urine. In time this can lead to damage to various organs including the eyes, kidneys and nervous system.

The disorder results from a deficiency or the diminished effectiveness of a hormone called insulin which is present

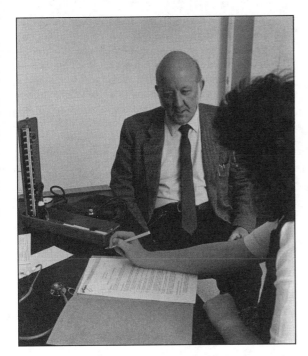

Figure 2.1 Robert Lawson consults his doctor: 'I've been getting these pains in my legs....'

in normal people. A hormone is a chemical that circulates in the bloodstream and influences the functioning of cells throughout the body. Insulin is produced by special glands in the pancreas, an organ in the abdomen, and is involved in regulating the uptake of sugar from the blood into muscles and other body organs.

Two main types of diabetes mellitus have been identified — Type I (also known as juvenile-onset or insulin-dependent diabetes) and Type II (also referred to as maturity-onset or non-insulin-dependent). Type I usually starts in childhood or adolescence. It seems that because of their genetic makeup some people are more likely to develop it than others. However, it also appears that some environmental factor (virus infections and emotional upsets have been suggested) is necessary to precipitate the disease. In Type II the genetic influence is even greater than in Type I. Type II is also associated with obesity.

The treatment of diabetes may involve dietary changes, or drugs taken by mouth that lower the level of sugar in the blood, or insulin injections. The choice of which treatment/s to use depends on the kind of diabetes a person is thought to be suffering from. However, all diabetics have to observe careful dietary control: over-eating will cause the blood sugar level to go too high (hyperglycaemia); on the other hand, if people receiving insulin injections do not eat enough there may be a dramatic fall in the blood sugar level (hypoglycaemia) culminating in the person passing into a coma.

Finally, it must be pointed out that there is another condition, called diabetes insipidus, which is now recognised as a completely separate disease from diabetes mellitus. It is characterised by the passing of large quantities of dilute urine as a result of a deficiency of a hormone called antidiuretic hormone. Compared with diabetes mellitus it is a rare condition. Any references to 'diabetes' in this book will always mean the common condition, diabetes mellitus.

We have described the idealised medical consultation to illustrate the main components of what is known as the *clinical method*; that is, the method used by doctors and others engaged in clinical work, whether they be heart surgeons or school health nurses, to decide what (if anything) is medically wrong with a person and what the appropriate corrective action should be.

The first step in the application of the clinical method is inevitably the patient's presentation to the doctor of a complaint or *symptom*.

☐ Can you suggest some common symptoms?
■ Pain, a skin rash, a lump, itching and weakness are some you may have thought of; there are many others.

It is important to recognise the difference between symptoms and diseases: any one of the symptoms listed could be a feature of several diseases, from the common and trivial to the rare and life-threatening. The clinical method is employed to distinguish between such alternatives. In the consultation described, the symptom Mr Lawson presented to his doctor was pain in his legs.

☐ What happened next in the consultation, and why?
■ The doctor sought more detailed information about the nature, severity and frequency of the pain (such as how often it occurred and where in his legs it was worst). This information helped the doctor to get a clearer picture of the main symptom — the first step towards drawing up a list of possible reasons for the leg pains.

In addition, the doctor asked about other aspects of Mr Lawson's health. In other words, she did not rely on Mr Lawson having volunteered everything that might be relevant. In the event, the need to pass urine at night proved to be particularly important in directing the doctor's attention — a symptom that Mr Lawson had not considered relevant to his present concern, leg pains. Thus, the second stage of the clinical method involves the doctor *taking a history* of the patient's past and present health.

☐ Why do you think the doctor asked about Mr Lawson's work and home life?
■ She may have been considering either a psychological basis for Mr Lawson's symptoms (such as a threat of redundancy or marital difficulties), or she may have been checking on the possibility that he might have been exposed to some toxic substance at work.

At this point in the consultation the doctor has to decide what diseases might be responsible for these symptoms. Sometimes this is straightforward. For instance, if Mr Lawson had been hit by a car then the cause of his painful legs would have been obvious, and the doctor would have been able to move on immediately to considering treatment. But sometimes there may be dozens of possible diseases to consider. The range of possibilities is referred to as the *differential diagnosis*, from which the eventual diagnosis will be selected.

The next stage in the clinical method is to test these possible diagnoses in the hope of disproving all but one.

☐ How did the doctor approach this in the consultation?
■ She acquired further information, first by examining the patient and then by carrying out various investigations.

The purpose of examination in the clinical method is to elicit *signs* of disease. Signs are what doctors see or feel when they carry out a physical examination; symptoms are the problems patients complain about. In our example, the doctor examined Mr Lawson's legs for signs of varicose veins, checked the pulses to assess the blood supply (an impaired supply could cause pain), tested his reflexes and whether he could sense vibration (both diminished or lost in diabetes) and examined his eyes (for other signs of diabetes). The signs revealed by these examinations all pointed to a *diagnosis* of diabetes. The doctor sought further support for what she believed to be the probable diagnosis by performing various investigations. She was not prepared to tell Mr Lawson that diabetes was the cause until she had obtained confirmation from these tests. And indeed her diagnosis was confirmed.

The diagnosis leads on to the two final stages of the clinical method — *treatment* and *prognosis*. The choice of treatment is based on two factors: the views currently held by the medical profession and the personal judgement of the doctor involved. In other words, although there is a generally accepted body of clinical knowledge, individual doctors may hold different opinions and beliefs about the 'correct' action to take. Some treatments are so well established that there is little or no variation in the therapy recommended by different doctors. Thus, if Mr Lawson's diabetes had first become apparent as a coma resulting from hyperglycaemia (a very high level of sugar in the blood), then there would have been no variation among doctors in the treatment he would have received — they would all have agreed to give him a life-saving injection of insulin. However, given the way he did in fact present his symptoms, such a uniform response would be most unlikely. Some doctors would suggest a change in diet, others would prescribe tablets or insulin, and yet others would opt for various combinations of treatment.

☐ Can you suggest why such variation in clinical decision-making may exist?

■ There are two main reasons. The first is the lack of scientific evaluation of the effectiveness of the different treatments available; that is, it is not known which is the most effective one. The second reason is doctors' defence of 'clinical freedom'.

The concept of clinical freedom — freedom to consider each person's illness as unique and therefore to some extent in need of an individualised decision about the 'correct' treatment — is a key topic in any consideration of health care.*

The prognosis, the likely future for the patient in terms of length of life and symptoms, is more difficult for the doctor to determine. It depends on the stage the disease has

reached, on the likely effect of the treatment, and on the patient's own psychological response, both to the diagnosis of the disease and to its treatment. In addition, a prognosis can only ever be an *average* assessment; so inevitably it will be an underestimate for some and an overestimate for others.

Despite the simplified nature of this account of the clinical method, it demonstrates two important aspects of the approach — the clinical (or medical) concept of *causation*, and the view of ill-health as a collection of discrete '*diseases*'. When the doctor tells Mr Lawson that his leg pains are 'caused' by diabetes, she is using the term 'cause' in a particular medical way. She means that certain symptoms are caused by a specific disease. Similarly, doctors talk of chest pain being caused by a heart attack and swollen, painful joints being caused by arthritis. This is a fairly limited use of the concept of causation. In essence, all that doctors are doing is to tell their patient the disease label for their illness. Of course, within the notion of a 'disease' is an explanation of the cause. As you have seen, for diabetes it is a lack of insulin.

Those trained in other methodologies might answer the question 'What is the cause of Mr Lawson's leg pains?' in rather different ways. Biologists might point out the strong genetic and familial factors and environmental influences such as viral infections; social scientists might be more concerned with why Mr Lawson was overweight (a factor that may be associated with the development of diabetes) and with the psychological and socioeconomic conditions associated with an increased likelihood of developing the condition. In other words, each discipline has its own concept of causality which reflects its own perspective. Before considering these non-clinical views in greater detail, we should discuss further the clinical notion of 'disease' and the uses and limitations of the clinical method.

What are 'diseases'?

We have seen how the clinical method depends on the existence of a body of medical knowledge that categorises states of ill-health into discrete 'diseases' such as diabetes, atherosclerosis (degeneration of the arteries leading to impaired blood flow) and varicose veins. Each disease label refers to a pattern of factors that occur in many people in more or less the same way. An American doctor, Lester King, described this process in a paper published in the 1950s.

... pain in the right lower quadrant of the abdomen, with nausea, vomiting, a fever, and a high white [cell] count, spell out the features of acute appendicitis ... a condition of fever, cough, runny nose, sore eyes, and the later appearance of characteristic spots on the skin, we call measles. Each of these diseases, so called,

---

* Clinical freedom is discussed in greater detail in *Caring for Health: Dilemmas and Prospects*. The Open University (1985) *Caring for Health: Dilemmas and Prospects*, The Open University Press. (U205 *Health and Disease*, Book VIII)

is a congeries [aggregation] of factors, and no single
factor, by itself, identifies the disease. It is only
the recurrence of a pattern of events, a number
of elements combined in a definite relationship,
which we can label a disease. (King, 1954, p.197)

The identification and distinguishing of different diseases
is therefore crucial to the success of the clinical method.
The difficulty this can present has long been recognised.
Elisha Bartlett, a doctor writing in 1844, talked of how
diseases may: '... approach and touch each other in so
many respects, and at so many points, that it may not be
possible, always in the present state of our knowledge, to
fix upon positive means for distinguishing between them.'
(quoted in King, 1954, p.198) This is as true today as in the
mid-nineteenth century. The 'discovery' of new diseases is
often simply the realisation that what has been considered
a single disease is in fact two or more. A recent example is
the 'discovery' of Legionnaires' disease — a type of
pneumonia which had not previously been distinguished
from other forms of pneumonia.

The categorisation of illness into diseases changes over
time. Indeed Lester King has gone so far as to suggest that
'the history of medicine is the history of distinguishing one
condition from another'. Historical examples abound, for
example the separation of smallpox from measles.*

Given that the categorisation of disease is constantly
changing as symptoms and signs are regrouped, we need to
consider how these definitions actually arise. Lester King
regards the identification of diseases as the result of the
work of individual clinicians. 'The great men in medicine
are those who can perceive similarities, patterns, relationships, and a "belonging together" of seemingly quite
discrete factors.' (King, 1954, p.198) The emphasis on the
importance of individuals to medical progress reflects the
traditional historical view of the progress of medicine and
science. However, by concentrating on the contribution of
individuals, this view ignores the work of others in the same
field of enquiry, the social and economic circumstances that
made research feasible, and the attitudes and beliefs of the
contemporary society which accommodated the new
ideas.†

One of the first 'great men' in medicine was Thomas
Sydenham (1624–89) who believed that the patterns of
illness he and others described, reflected a natural order
similar to the classification of plant species into hierarchies

of related types (another major concern of seventeenth-
century and eighteenth-century science). Sydenham argued
that clinicians could escape from the apparent chaos of
illnesses in all their various forms, and discover clear
patterns of diseases. Such faith in the idea of a natural order
of diseases turned out to be overly optimistic. The changing
nature of disease categories and definitions (e.g. diabetes,
discussed below) is evidence of the absence of such absolute
patterns. It is often difficult for us to recognise diseases
from the descriptions of clinicians in the past. However,
there are some notable exceptions, such as Hippocrates'
description of mumps dating from around 400 BC, which is
still apt today. The classification of diseases is not simply
of historical interest however. A leading British psychi-
atrist, David Goldberg, has recently called for a new
taxonomy (or classification) based on the types of
psychological disorders seen by general practitioners who
'have the greatest difficulty in assimilating their patients
who have subtle combinations of physical symptoms and
emotional problems'.

Much of the reason for alterations in disease categories
arises from changes in the criteria for defining diseases.
Diabetes provides a good example of this. The name comes
from the Greek word for 'a passer through, a siphon' — a
description of the main symptoms of drinking and
urinating large volumes. In the eighteenth century William
Cullen (1710–90) in his study of diseases, *Nosologia*,
described diabetes as 'the pissing evile', characterised by
'the immoderate discharge of urine, in general unlike the
natural; of long continuance'. Diabetes was subdivided into
diabetes mellitus, 'with urine the smell, colour and taste of
honey', and diabetes insipidus, 'with limpid urine not
sweet'. Nowadays, these two 'subdivisions' are considered
to be completely separate diseases.

Over the past two centuries definitions of diseases have
shifted from the nature of the symptoms and signs, to the
underlying changes in the tissue — the pathology — and
from there to the chemistry of the cells and tissues.

☐   To illustrate how definitions of diseases evolve, try
to list the three stages in the definition of diabetes.

■   The stages were: (a) a description of the main
symptom — 'a siphon'; (b) a more detailed account
including the nature of the urine — the taste, smell and
appearance of the urine; and (c) a note of changes in the
chemistry of the body — that is in the level of the
hormone responsible for the disease (insulin).

In fact, recent developments in molecular biology have
taken the definition a stage further by describing the
biochemical characteristics of hormones. Thus the
categorisation of diseases can be seen to reflect the concerns
of clinical medicine and medical research at any particular
time. This is one reason why Sydenham's hopes could not

---

* There are further examples in *Medical Knowledge: Doubt and
Certainty* and *The Health of Nations*. The Open University (1985)
Medical Knowledge: Doubt and Certainty, The Open University
Press. The Open University (1985) *The Health of Nations*, The
Open University Press. (U205 *Health and Disease*, Books II and III)
† These issues will be discussed further in *Medical Knowledge:
Doubt and Certainity*.

be realised. This account should also caution us against adhering too strongly to our own definitions and categories of disease, as pointed out by Lester King:

> As we, in our own experience, create one pattern after another, we wonder whether these match the patterns of Reality. Sometimes we feel that we have constructed a reasonable approximation. Then we can only wait and see how our proffered blueprint of organisation enables us to deal with future experience. Our difficulties arise only when we are arrogant in our assurance. (King, 1954, p.203)

Before we leave this issue it should be noted that prevailing theories not only influence the work of clinicians but also our own behaviour as patients, as explained in a recent description by an American doctor, Tristram Engelhardt:

> ... theories tell clinicians what to look for, what to ignore, and what to act upon. Of course, they also tell patients what to see, for patients are schooled both directly and indirectly in the realities of illness and of medical disorders. As a result, given different background assumptions, different things will stand out in the patient's experience of his or her illness. In short prevailing biomedical viewpoints fashion the life-world of patients so that their disorders appear already shaped in part by scientific understandings of disease. (Engelhardt, 1981, p.305)

What is disease?

We have seen how clinical observations have led doctors to define and redefine diseases, but we have not yet considered how a particular set of experiences is first designated as a diseased state (rather than a healthy one) and therefore warranting medical categorisation. In other words, what is *disease*? Such considerations are not of purely philosophical interest. It is important to the study of health and disease to appreciate that the designation 'diseased' is to some extent arbitrary, being influenced by social and cultural factors. This can best be seen by considering ways in which we can attempt to define the term 'disease'. Before reading on, try to construct a definition of 'disease' for yourself.

Various approaches to this question have been adopted. These can be grouped broadly into those in which some objective scientific measurement is used (often referred to as the *biomedical approach*) such as the use of blood sugar levels in diabetes, and those based on *self-assessment*, the person's subjective assessment of how they feel. Both approaches present particular difficulties.

The biomedical approach can be based on a statistical definition of disease (which will be discussed in later chapters). For example, diabetics have been defined as

people with a level of sugar in their blood in excess of a particular value (about the equivalent of one gram of glucose per litre of blood) after fasting for several hours. However, a few people have levels above this, but show no symptoms or signs of 'disease'. Should we consider them to be 'diseased' and try to treat them?

There are also difficulties in defining 'diseased' on the basis of a person's subjective assessment. First, a claim such as 'I feel fine' may not be entirely reliable as the person may actually be harbouring a symptomless form of diabetes that may result in blindness in the not-too-distant future. Second, such a model depends on the person's expectation of health — if you do not expect to be able to run at the age of 57 then inability to do so will not be seen as unhealthy. Conversely, pain, discomfort, and disability may not always be associated with disease; for example, infants who are teething or women in labour both suffer pain. Our view of disease reflects the prevailing cultural attitudes. Lester King gives the example of foot-binding in China in which women suffered pain and disability but were not considered diseased.

You will be learning more about definitions of health and disease, but at this stage it is enough to realise that this subject is problematic, and that neither the biomedical approach, nor subjective assessments provide completely adequate definitions. In practice we need to adopt an approach that encompasses both, such as that suggested by Lester King: 'Disease is the aggregate of those conditions which, judged by the prevailing culture, are deemed painful, or disabling, and which at the same time, deviate from either the statistical norm or from some idealised status.' (King, 1954, p.197) We come back to just what might be meant by the 'statistical norm' in later chapters.

The uses and limitations of the clinical method

Having discussed the concepts on which the clinical method is based, it is necessary to consider the two purposes for which it is used — the management of individual problems and the study of disease.

In the first part of this chapter, a typical medical consultation was described. Because we simplified it to highlight the components of the clinical method you may have gained the impression that the diagnosis of disease is without problems. This is far from true. Three problems in particular need mentioning: (a) the dominance of disease definitions; (b) the reliability of the method; and (c) clinical judgement. We have already seen how definitions of disease influence what clinicians look for and how patients may present their problems. This may affect all stages of the method — history-taking, examination and investigation. The dominance of the notion of discrete diseases means that clinicians attempt to fit patients' problems to one such label. In many cases this is of benefit to the patient.

However, there is a risk of *inappropriate labelling* which may be difficult to remove. Richard Asher, a doctor writing in the 1960s, described how this may arise:

> We shut our eyes to observations which do not agree with the conclusions we wish to reach. We close our ears to bits of history which seem out of place, or to noises coming down our stethoscopes which are not included in the catalogue of official sounds we have been taught to recognise. (Asher, 1972, p.2)

A second difficulty is the *reliability of the clinical method*. Skilled physicians examining a patient may disagree about what they find. In the example consultation, the doctor checked for the presence of arterial pulses in Mr Lawson's legs — a procedure you may consider straightforward. However, a study of this procedure found that three physicians disagreed in 31 per cent of examinations as to whether or not a pulse was present in the feet.

The importance of the third problem — *clinical judgement* — is best explained by an example. A group of several hundred children complaining of recurrent tonsillitis was seen by a surgeon. Half of them were judged as needing surgery. The other half were seen by another surgeon (who did not know they had already been turned down for surgery) and of these half were judged as needing the operation. The remaining children were taken to another surgeon, who also recommended half for surgery. You may find this incredible, amusing or horrifying. The important point to note is that clinical judgement (like other aspects of the clinical method) is largely based on the clinicians' belief about what will most benefit the patient, rather than on scientific knowledge.

Apart from its use in diagnosis, the clinical method is also used in the study of health and disease. There have been some notable successes from two related methods of enquiry — the case study and the case series. The *case study* is, as the name suggests, a detailed study of a particular case of ill-health (i.e. of an individual patient). Paul Beeson, a leading contemporary United States physician, considers some of medicine's best achievements have begun with such bedside observations. In support of this he gives the example of leucine (a substance found in cow's milk) and seizures in infants: 'the discovery that leucine causes hypoglycaemia [low blood sugar levels] was made because a paediatrician observed that an infant had seizures more frequently when fed cow's milk than when breast-fed.' (Beeson, 1977, p.2209)

□ Can you suggest what the main limitation of the case-study approach might be?

■ It is good at detecting the odd, unusual, rare associations, but not very effective at spotting common associations.

Identifying common associations is just what the *case series* can achieve. By observing a number of individuals with the same condition, the alert clinician may notice some factor common to all of them. In the 1950s it was noted that several people suffering from nasopharyngeal cancer (at the back of the nasal cavity) had been employed as woodworkers. Further research confirmed a causal relationship; material the woodworkers were handling was causing these cancers. The case-series method requires even greater powers of observation than the case study. The difference between the methods has been likened to the difference between noticing a parrot on a suburban bird-table (the rare, unusual observation of the case study) and noticing twice the usual number of sparrows (a change in the quantity of a common, frequently-made observation).

Despite the successes of these methods both are inevitably limited by their restricted field of view — 'the diseased'. In addition, these methods are by definition confined to clinical settings — hospital wards, outpatient departments and clinics. Such environments can have a marked effect on people's behaviour. However, it is perhaps another aspect of the clinical method that represents its most serious limitation — its strict adherence to an established categorisation of diseases. This danger has been described by Richard Asher:

> We refrain from speaking about things that we observe when they are not listed in the official phenomena of the text-book description; apart from that we refrain from speaking our own opinions when they conflict too violently with generally accepted thought, or when they are greatly at variance with the opinions of those we fear. It is probably to our advantage that we do so, but it is of no advantage to the forward march of medical science.
> (Asher, 1972, p.2)

Finally, the clinical method is inevitably limited in its ability to determine the underlying causes of diseases — factors that will lie far outside the confines of the clinical setting. This can only be achieved by methods used by the natural and social sciences. The role of the clinical method in *studying* disease (as distinct from treating it) is to make observations and pose questions for these other disciplines to investigate. Before we consider their methodologies, a final comment on the importance of the clinical method from Paul Beeson: 'Clinicians have made and will continue to make fundamental contributions to biologic [sic] thought. The best clinical investigation deserves to rank as a science along with any of the other disciplines. Observations made at the bedside have often contributed substantial new insight into the basic sciences.' (Beeson, 1977, p.2209)

Objectives for Chapter 2

When you have studied this chapter, you should be able to:

2.1 Describe (in your own words) the features of the clinical method including the meaning of symptoms, signs, differential diagnosis, diagnosis, treatment and prognosis.

2.2 Describe what doctors mean by 'a disease'; explain how particular disease categories arise; and why such categories change over time.

2.3 Explain what is meant by 'disease', the difference between objective and subjective explanations of disease and why the term is difficult to define.

2.4 Contrast the two clinical approaches to the study of health and disease — the case study and the case series — and describe their methodological limitations.

Questions for Chapter 2

1 (*Objective 2.1*) Is each of (a)–(f) a symptom, a sign or a disease?
- (a) pneumonia
- (b) a cough first thing in the morning
- (c) an enlarged liver
- (d) a sore throat
- (e) enlarged tonsils
- (f) tonsillitis

2 (*Objective 2.2*) Over the past few decades the number of people certified as dying from coronary heart disease (heart attacks) has substantially increased, whereas deaths from a condition called myocardial degeneration (degeneration of the heart) have decreased. From what you have read in this chapter, what explanation can you offer for these changes?

3 (*Objective 2.3*) Suppose your doctor decided to check all the people registered with his or her practice for sugar in their urine and found that yours was abnormal despite the fact that you felt well. Would you then be 'healthy' or would you have a disease?

4 (*Objective 2.4*) A new washing-powder comes on the market. Within a few weeks people are claiming that it causes skin rashes. Which method — case study or case series — would be more useful in establishing support for this claim?

3

Biological approaches to health and disease

When you have finished working through Chapter 2, you should have been convinced that medical diagnosis is a complex business. The definitions of disease and decisions about appropriate treatments are not fixed but fluctuate with the state of scientific knowledge, with social expectation and with the state of medical opinion or fashion at any time. The consultation between the doctor and Robert Lawson involved a complex interaction in which Mr Lawson described ways in which he felt pain, or was not his 'normal self'. Prompted by the doctor he went on to discuss other aspects of his condition that might be considered important. The doctor based her questions on past experience of other patients and on what the text-books and medical school training had indicated as possibly important symptoms. She then moved on to the next step, making measurements. Mr Lawson's eyes were examined with an ophthalmoscope, his urine was tested for sugar.

By this time, the doctor had made a *hypothesis* (an informed guess) about the cause of Mr Lawson's pains and was testing that hypothesis by measurement. If there were sugar in Mr Lawson's urine, this would tend to confirm the doctor's hypothesis that the patient was suffering from diabetes. If the blood sugar level were 'normal', then the diabetes hypothesis would be improbable, and some other explanation would have to be sought.

This making and testing of hypotheses is essentially the model on which so-called *scientific medicine* is based. It assumes that: (a) an individual's pain or distress arises from a malfunctioning of some aspect of the working of their body, that is from their biology; (b) this malfunction can be detected by making measurements of the workings of the body (for instance, feeling for arterial pulses in Mr Lawson's legs or studying the back of his eyes with an ophthalmoscope or measuring the sugar level in his blood); and (c) when the malfunction has been detected it can be

In this chapter we refer to a number of biological methods, approaches and concepts. You need to understand them only insofar as they relate to the chapter's objectives and help to illuminate what we refer to as the biomedical approach. They are discussed more fully in Book IV, *The Biology of Health and Disease*, and, in some instances, Book VI, *Experiencing and Explaining Disease*.

At the end of Chapter 3 we ask you to turn to Book II, *Medical Knowledge: Doubt and Certainty*, which places the traditional biomedical approach to health and disease in a wider context, and thus demonstrates its limitations. Book II will set today's knowledge of health and disease in a wide social and historical context, showing how concepts of what constitutes health and what is an appropriate treatment for disease vary in different cultures and in western society over the past several centuries. This will move the focus of your study from individuals to the investigation of groups and of society in general, which is the substance of Chapters 4–12 of this book.

treated in some way by administering chemicals (drugs) or other treatment to the patient. In this way either the pain or distress resulting from the disease can be reduced or the malfunction can actually be corrected; for instance, the symptoms of Mr Lawson's diabetes can be corrected by adjusting the level of the body chemical insulin (a hormone) in the bloodstream. This approach to the treatment of Mr Lawson is what is referred to in the previous chapter as the *biomedical approach*.

This may all seem very obvious, but this 'scientific' view of the medical process is itself a relatively recent development and is historically linked to the development of ideas about science in general as a way of exploring, explaining and transforming the world, which we shall discuss in Chapters 11 and 12. By locating the 'cause' of Mr Lawson's illness in his biology, scientific medicine rules out (or seems to rule out) other explanations: for example, that it is a normal part of Mr Lawson's life experience and does not require to be specially accounted for; that it is a punishment by God for some misdeed or the result of witchcraft by some ill-wisher; that it is a manifestation of his psychological state; or a consequence of economic factors or poor working conditions. We shall return later to how these different explanations might be related. For the moment, we are concerned to explore a little further the implications and assumptions of these biological approaches to understanding the pains with which Mr Lawson is afflicted.

Studying disease in humans

Scientific medicine is, then, based on (and in its turn offers) an understanding of the biology of humans. How can biological knowledge of humans be obtained? The starting point is always *observation*. Traditional medicine, which in Western societies extends from ancient times through to the eighteenth and nineteenth centuries, relied on *empirical* remedies, that is remedies based on practice, trial and error and accumulated experience, such as knowledge of the beneficial effects of particular extracts of plants or animals — the starting point for many present-day drugs. Or it practised intervention, such as blood-letting, by opening veins or applying leeches, for almost any type of disorder.

Modern scientific medicine came about with the development of the so-called 'scientific method' of making hypotheses and testing them by experimentation, which took place in Europe from the seventeenth century onwards. It was then that the systematic exploration of the human body by dissection of cadavers (human corpses) and the testing of living people began. Dissection is the starting point for *anatomy*, the study of body structures. Tests on the properties of living bodies, for instance on the contraction of muscles or the beating of the heart, are the starting point for *physiology*. Tests on the composition of

blood, its sugar content, for instance, are the starting point for *biochemistry*, the chemistry of life. Even before these new biological sciences began to develop, the methods of observation and empirical treatment of human disease began to yield dramatic successes.

In fact, the history of medicine and the history of biology have been intertwined from the very beginning. Biological research did not become the vast scientific enterprise that it is today merely as a result of the abstract search for 'knowledge for its own sake'. True, it arose in part from people's curiosity about the living world around them and the part their own bodies played in life's processes. But it was also driven by the very practical needs of agriculture — how best to plant and harvest crops and improve livestock yields — and of medicine — how to cure the ills of the human body. Indeed much biological research continues to be 'driven' by medical questions today, as it was in the seventeenth century. The search for a 'cure for cancer' leads biologists to explore questions of cell growth and division.* The apparently endless hunt for new drugs leads to esoteric research on the interactions between complex artificially synthesised chemicals and the myriad chemical reactions that go on constantly within the cells of the body. But for much of the history of biology, medical interests have been firmly in the driving seat.

For instance, sailors on long voyages frequently suffered a disease called scurvy, characterised by bleeding gums, loosened teeth and slow healing of wounds. In the 1750s, during Captain Cook's naval expedition to Australia, citrus fruits and fresh vegetables were added to the diet of sailors on board ship and the result was that scurvy was either prevented or cured (thereby accidentally rediscovering something the Chinese had known 200 years previously). By 1800, British sailors were being issued routinely with lemon and lime juice on long voyages, although the biochemical reasons for the effectiveness of the citrus fruits were not known until the twentieth century. (They contain ascorbic acid, or vitamin C, which is necessary for many cellular processes to occur, but which the human body cannot manufacture.)

Similarly, in the 1770s a country doctor, Edward Jenner, drew a crucial medical conclusion from the folk knowledge that villagers who had suffered from the mild disease of cowpox seemed not to catch the much more serious smallpox; and introduced the now famous technique of

---

* The relevance of cell growth and cell division to cancer and its treatment is discussed in *The Biology of Health and Disease* and *Experiencing and Explaining Disease*. The Open University (1985) *The Biology of Health and Disease*, The Open University Press. The Open University (1985) *Experiencing and Explaining Disease*, The Open University Press. (U205 *Health and Disease*, Books IV and VI).

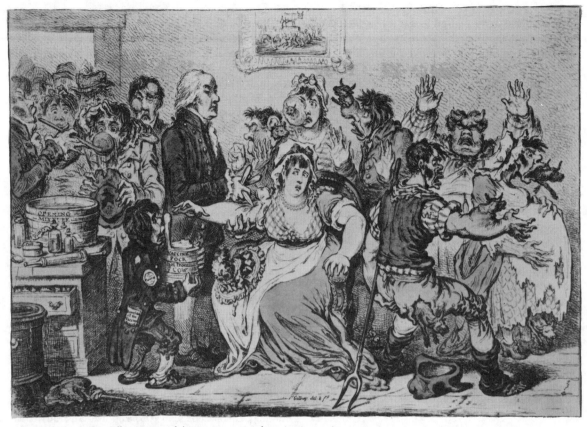

Figure 3.1 Cartoonist Gillray's view of the consequences of vaccination against cowpox.

vaccination — injecting a healthy person with a solution containing the cowpox-producing agent — which has formed the prototype for all subsequent immunisation programmes.

These are examples of how observation, followed by the systematic trial of proposed remedies, can lead to effective treatments for disease. Perhaps one of the best examples comes from the disease, pellagra, known for centuries to be *endemic* (that is, constantly present) among the poor. Pellagra is characterised by rough red skin, eruptions, diarrhoea, lassitude, dizziness and various mental disorders ranging from depression to violent lunacy. By the early twentieth century, pellagra was recognised as a major scourge among the poor of the southern states of the USA. But what caused it? There was no lack of hypotheses: eating too much of the wrong sort of corn; the presence of infectious microorganisms, or parasites; the side-effects of syphilis; or the genetically weak constitution held to prevail among the very poor. Yet no amount of drugging, with those chemicals that were available at the time, could cure the disease. The classic proof of the cause of pellagra was made by Joseph Goldberger, an epidemiologist, between

1914 and 1920. He began with noting the distribution of pellagra in the community — just who was affected and who was not. This approach, known as *epidemiology*, the study of patterns of disease, is discussed further in Chapter 6. Unlike typhus, or malaria, pellagra affected only the

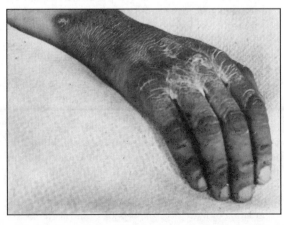

Figure 3.2 The rough, red skin that is typical of pellagra sufferers.

poor, and spared the rich. It affected the institutionalised — orphans, prisoners, inmates of mental asylums — but never their guardians. It affected mill-hands but never mill-owners.

□ What could this distribution of the disease indicate about how it was (or was not) transmitted?
■ It must mean that pellagra was not transmitted merely by contact between one person and another; that is, it was not a communicable disease.

Goldberger went on to prove this epidemiological conclusion in the most direct way possible. He and (later) other volunteers injected themselves with blood from a pellagra sufferer, and even went so far as to eat the skin scales and vomit of another. They did not contract the disease.

□ Try to construct a hypothesis about what could cause pellagra?
■ There must be something different about how the poor lived — and one obvious factor was what they ate.
□ How could one test this hypothesis?
■ By adding to the diet of the poor those things it characteristically lacked but were present in the diet of the rich — meat, dairy products, vegetables — one could test its validity.

Goldberger tested such additions to the diet of people in orphanages and asylums and found that pellagra could be cured speedily and eradicated. He deduced that these foods contained a substance, which he called a 'pellagra-preventative factor', that was necessary for health. Today it is called a vitamin (actually one of the vitamin B group). Finally, he did the 'experiment' the other, and most conclusive, way round.

□ What would that experiment involve?
■ It would involve removing the meat, etc. from the diet of people who did not have pellagra to see if they contracted the disease.

Goldberger persuaded a dozen Mississippi white convicts to live on a high starch diet with no protein or fresh green vegetables for six months. All showed signs of pellagra, and all were cured when protein and vegetables were reintroduced into the diet. (The ethics of this type of experiment is another question, to which we shall return in Chapter 6.)

The immediate *biological* cause of pellagra, and its cure (though not the biochemical nature of the preventive factor, nor how it actually worked), were then established beyond doubt by a combination of epidemiology, observation and direct experimentation on human subjects. However, the elimination of pellagra required (and still requires) not biological experimentation but social and economic change to eliminate the poverty that forces people to live on inadequate diets. For a complete description of the causes of pellagra, a definition of its biological causation is thus insufficient (Chapter 11).

The limitations of studying humans

How far can one locate the causes or cures of disease by studying humans? The first thing that is needed is a concept of what 'normal' healthy individuals are like — the range of their physiological and biochemical properties: the sound of their heartbeat, the characteristics of their pulse, the level of sugar in their blood, and so forth. Normal ranges may be rather broad (e.g. height) or narrow (e.g. body temperature, where fluctuation of no more than a degree or so away from the 'normal' point may be a symptom of illness). Abnormalities, defined either by rule of thumb (the doctor's experience), or by the statistical methods discussed in Chapter 5 then become of interest; an individual's 'high' temperature is high relative to their normal temperature, whereas 'high' blood sugar may be 'high' only relative to the average blood-sugar level for people of that sex and age group in the population (this was the way it was defined in Chapter 2 in relation to diabetes). On the other hand, not all abnormalities are of clinical interest. It is 'abnormal' for a man to be taller than, say, 2 metres (6′ 6″) in that very few men in Britain are that height, yet it is an abnormality that is of concern *mainly* when the man has to buy clothes or bend to go through doors (though it *could* be an indication of a hormonal imbalance). An adult's being shorter than, say 1.4 metres (4′ 7″) is, however, more likely to be of clinical interest. Definitions of abnormality are not absolute, but depend upon social expectations as much as upon formal statistics. (Recall the reference to foot-binding in Chapter 2.)

Studies of the distribution of disease within a population — its epidemiology — can be very revealing. For instance, it enables the two Types of diabetes to be distinguished.

□ Do you remember what the age distributions for the two Types were?
■ Broadly speaking, people with Type I are affected early in life whereas the onset of Type II tends to be in middle and old age.

One can go further, using such epidemiological methods, to learn something about biological causes of diseases. Pellagra turned out to be associated with a poor diet. But suppose it had turned out that it was concentrated in particular families, so that all the children of affected parents also showed the disease. The cause *might* be found in how a particular family lived — their environment — but you might also suspect that there could be another important cause.

☐ What might this cause be?

■ Children *inherit* an important part of their biology, their genes, from their parents. Could there be something in the genes of the parents and their children that was responsible for producing the disease?

There is a variety of ways of analysing for the possible genetic transmission of susceptibility to disease, based on looking at the distribution of the disease in individuals that are more or less closely related genetically. The relation of most genes to most diseases is extremely unclear. All body tissues are composed of cells, and each cell contains within it copies of the complete genetic material (the DNA) which provides the instructions for making the protein constituents of the cell. Each cell has some 10 million such different genes, though not all are 'used' by the cell.

There are some diseases that are the result of a single gene abnormality. Two examples are sickle cell anaemia and thalassaemia, blood diseases prevalent in people of African origin (sickle cell anaemia) and of Mediterranean origin (thalassaemia). But diabetes, like many other disorders, shows no such clear genetic association, though there is some evidence that genetic inheritance is one important factor, among others, in how likely a person is to develop the Type II diabetes. However, the effect is not strong, and clearly the environmental influences on a person as they develop are very important in determining whether or not an individual will show symptoms of diabetes that are worrying enough to make them consult a doctor.

There are a number of very new techniques becoming available to biology as a result of the development of what is known loosely as 'genetic engineering'. The use of such techniques enables individual human genes to be isolated, and there is as a result increasing knowledge of the properties of the genes that might be associated with diabetes.

So far as biologically based medicine is concerned, the distribution of a disease in the population and the surface properties of an individual sufferer — what we can measure in terms of blood pressure, temperature and so forth — are only the beginning of the study of normality and abnormality. Much is going on inside a person which may be important if it can be detected. Parts of the body are more available and accessible to analysis than others. The easiest of all are body fluids. For centuries medicine has examined urine, faeces (stools) and blood for abnormalities. Today another source of body fluid is also used — cerebrospinal fluid, the liquid inside the 'canal' that runs down the spine, which can be extracted by lumbar puncture (insertion of a needle into the lower back). Biopsies, small sections of tissue such as muscle or liver, are also sometimes

taken. Traditionally, doctors observed, smelt or tasted these materials. Such procedures, you will recall, led very early to the distinction between diabetes mellitus with 'sweet urine' and diabetes insipidus with 'limpid urine.' Today biologists separate their chemical constituents and perform automated chemical analyses on them.

'Abnormalities' can be revealing: sugar in the urine is a diagnostic sign for diabetes; abnormally high cholesterol (a fatty substance) in the blood may be associated with coronary heart disease; high levels of some proteins in the blood may indicate that the person has had a heart attack. But there is not always a simple relationship between the presence of a biological 'marker', such as cholesterol or sugar, and the clinical presence of disease. Many people with high blood cholesterol do not have heart attacks; mass-screening of the population for sugar in the urine reveals people who on this evidence alone would be classified as diabetic but who show none of the clinical signs of diabetes discussed in Chapter 2. The variability and interactions of human body chemistry are so rich that a direct equation of such-and-such a level of a particular chemical with the clinical signs of a disease is rarely certain.

What is more, if abnormal chemicals are found in body fluids or tissue derived from diseased persons, confusion of *cause* with *consequence* is easy. In the 1960s there were many reports that the urine of schizophrenic patients contained peculiar substances not seen in other patients. Could they be the mysterious 'cause' of schizophrenia? It turned out that the substances were chemical breakdown products of the drugs that were being administered to the schizophrenic individuals in hospital. When they were taken off the drugs, the substances disappeared from their urine. Even the fact that if people are depressed they may drink a lot of tea is likely to show up in the form of abnormal levels of substances such as the breakdown products of caffeine, tannin, and so forth, in their urine. The presence of such substances is a *consequence* of the illness, not a *cause* of it.

Trying to discover what is going on inside a person by analysing the food they eat or their blood or urine, is like trying to discover about the jobs and personal relationships of the dwellers in a house by looking at their grocery bills and digging around in their rubbish bins. One can learn a little — but one could be seriously misled.

The traditional answer of medical science to the question of finding out what is going on inside the person has been to wait until they are dead and then to cut them up — the *post-mortem study*. Post-mortems can often tell how a person died; they can say less about how they lived, or about how the disease they died of might be treated. Over the past few years a battery of new techniques for looking inside the living body has become available. These are based on the principle that although we cannot see

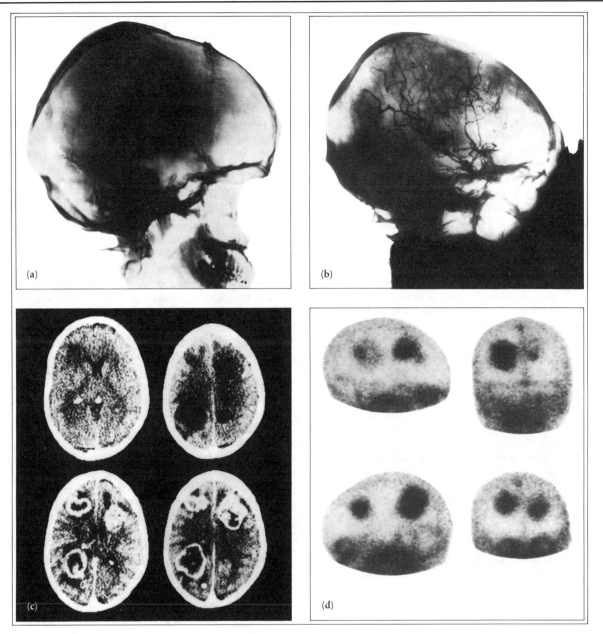

Figure 3.3 Four different ways of looking into a living body.

(a) 'Conventional' X-ray of the human head. The X-rays are stopped by the bony tissue and pass through the soft tissue. What you can see, therefore, is the shape of the bones.

(b) Angiogram of the head. To make this picture a substance that is opaque to X-rays is injected into the blood. This enables all the blood vessels as well as the skull to be seen.

(c) CT scan of the human brain. CT stands for computerised tomography. It uses an X-ray method but in a novel way: a narrow X-ray beam is shone through the head from multiple positions around the patient and the X-radiation transmitted to the other side of the body is measured. The many different pictures are combined by way of a computer, and a series of 'slices' through the brain can be studied. This enables abnormalities — perhaps associated with brain tumours, or with blocked blood vessels — to be located.

(d) Isotope scan. This is a way of measuring the distribution of specific substances — glucose, brain proteins or whatever — inside the head of a living subject. Specific radioactively labelled substances (the actual dose is equivalent to about ten chest X-rays) are injected into the bloodstream. Computerised tomography, as in (b), enables concentrations of these substances to be localised to particular brain regions.

directly into the body, because it is opaque to visible light, other forms of radiation can pass through at least the soft tissue of the body. The oldest of such procedures is the X-ray, which passes short-wavelength radiation through the body. The rays traverse the soft tissues easily, but are stopped by bones. Other body organs can be made radio-opaque (for instance the stomach and gut can be made radio-opaque by eating food containing barium chloride) and can also be photographed with X-rays. Newer types of scanner (e.g. so-called CT scans — CT stands for computerised tomography) work on the same principle but use computers to analyse the results. Another method involves injecting (harmless) radioactive substances into the bloodstream, which can 'map' the blood circulation and show up blockages or tumours — particularly useful in studying the brain. Ultrasound (high-frequency sound waves) can be used to monitor the size of the unborn baby in the womb, because the waves are reflected to different degrees by body tissues of different densities. And the latest methods at the time of writing make use of giant magnetic fields to measure the internal chemistry of the body and the functioning of its organs.

Scanners, the biochemical analysis of body fluids and even the most sophisticated genetic analysis go only so far. It is a basic principle of the biomedical model that if you really want to discover the biological cause of a phenomenon occurring in any living creature, then you must take the organism apart, intervene in its normal working, experiment on it. This was Goldberger's approach to pellagra, for instance. The limitations of what can be achieved by such approaches in humans are partly ethical, but only partly. There is a limit to what even the most 'heroic' of researchers can discover by researching on their own bodies. Hence the need to find substitutes for humans on which to practice intervention, test theories, or discover fundamental biological properties.

From humans to other animals

Albrecht von Haller, a leading eighteenth-century physiologist, wrote:

> It is not sufficient to make dissections of the dead bodies of animals. It is necessary to incise them in the living state. There is no action in the dead body; all movement must be studied in the living animal and the whole of physiology turns on the motions, external and internal of the living body ... a single experiment will sometimes refute years of speculation.

The essential features of investigative natural science are first, observation, then making hypotheses about the world, then systematic intervention into the objects that are being studied, and examination of the results of such interventions. That is what *experiments* are about.

As you saw in Chapter 2, there has been a long history of research into diabetes and its origins. But understanding what *caused* diabetes required more than just observation and tasting urine. In 1889, in Strasbourg, Oscar Minkowski and Josef von Mehring found that removing the pancreas of a dog produced diabetes in the animal. The pancreas is a large glandular organ located close to the stomach, whose main function was already known to be the secretion of certain digestive juices into the gut. So could something present in the pancreas alleviate the disease? Simply mincing up the pancreas and feeding it to diabetics did not work. But in Toronto between 1920 and 1922 the young surgeon Frederick Banting and his colleague Charles Best, a medical student, tied up the pancreatic ducts of dogs, thus allowing the secreted juices to accumulate. Eventually they were able to collect enough pancreatic secretions first to show that they could keep diabetic dogs alive and later to inject into diabetic patients. When injected into a patient the juice did indeed prevent the excretion of sugar in the urine. Chemical purification of the juice enabled a protein to be extracted, which had the same properties as the pancreatic juice: it enabled the body to use the sugar, rather than to excrete it. The protein was called insulin. The point is that without experimental intervention no amount of observation of human sufferers would have given the information that the experiment on dogs produced. (There is another important lesson in the insulin story. To move from laboratory experiment to the production of a substance in bulk for use in human patients required, very early on, the involvement of industry. Banting's Professor, J. J. R. Macleod, brought the US drug company Eli Lilly into the collaboration, and Lilly has been one of the world's major producers of insulin ever since.)

The biology of other mammals is reasonably similar to the biology of humans. Their internal organs are arranged similarly; they react similarly to many chemicals and drugs; their bodies, if injured, heal according to similar mechanisms; they are subject to many of the same diseases — some 60 per cent of human diseases have analogues in dogs for instance. These similarities depend upon the extraordinary biochemical and cellular similarities that run through the entire living world. The basic principles of the organisation of life are the same for human or non-human animals — and indeed for plants and bacteria. Hence, medical research can make use of so-called 'animal models' in studying human biology in health and disease.

An 'animal model' in this sense is a system that may be either a simplified version of the 'real thing' or one that is available for and amenable to experimental manipulation. The closer the non-human animal is to humans in evolutionary terms, the better a model it becomes. The closest living relative to *Homo sapiens* is the chimpanzee; it has over 98 per cent of its genes in common with humans.

Other mammals are further apart from us in their biology. None the less, studying them can provide reliable information about human biology. In diabetes, the organ whose failure resulted in the disease was shown to be the pancreas by the use of dogs, and potential treatments for diabetics, such as the feeding of pancreatic extract, could be tested out in dogs. Today, research on insulin and its metabolism (its chemical and cellular interactions with body tissue) continues on experimental animals. Diabetes can be induced in them surgically, by the removal of the pancreas, and also, today, by specific drugs that prevent the production of insulin.

Disease and treatments of disease can be explored in animals in ways that would be ethically impossible in humans. But there are many who argue that we should not be doing experiments on animals at all. Although humans must exploit other life forms to survive, as we need at least to eat plants, not being able to derive our biochemical energy any other way, it would be possible to survive without eating, exploiting, or experimenting on other animals. One does not have to be a vegan to recognise that there may be acceptable alternatives to some forms of animal experimentation; if we lived in a society that generated fewer new types of chemicals and was less drug-oriented, fewer safety tests would be required. For some types of use of animals other alternatives might be devised — experiments with single-celled organisms (which few people would object to) or with cultures of cells, for instance. But for many uses of animals for *medical* research it remains difficult to see an effective alternative: the question that must then be answered is: is there an overriding loyalty to the human species that justifies the exploitation of non-human creatures? It is up to you to answer *that* question according to your own lights.

From animals to atoms

The nearest animal model to the human is clearly another large animal. But general principles of body physiology can be studied in other kinds of animals — birds, fish, frogs or even animals without backbones (non-vertebrates). Valuable information about body chemistry can be obtained even from such microscopic, single-celled organisms as yeasts and bacteria. Nor does the living animal always have to be used. If tissue is removed from an animal, say a piece of liver, and then slices are cut from it and bathed in a warm solution containing oxygen and sugar, the cells of the slice will go on working biochemically for several hours, enabling many fundamental cellular properties to be explored. Such slices will 'burn' sugar to provide energy, and give off carbon dioxide; they will synthesise proteins and lipids (fats) and perform some of the 'physiological' functions of the organ from which they have been taken

— for instance, secreting hormones if a gland; contracting if a muscle; and so forth. Thus the effects of insulin in the 'medium' surrounding such slices can be studied with great precision.

If a tissue slice is broken up gently — for instance by rubbing though a nylon cloth or by the use of particular chemicals — the individual cells of which it is composed can be separated. The cells from some types of tissue can be settled onto a glass plate, and under appropriate conditions will begin to grow and multiply. Such 'tissue cultures' can be kept alive for many days. Some types of culture, derived from cancer tissue, become to all intents and purposes immortal; the cells can be kept growing and multiplying indefinitely. Again, biochemical experiments or explorations of the effects of drugs can be conducted upon such tissue cultures.

Slices of tissue derived from organs, cells derived from them and single-celled creatures such as yeast and bacteria are all clearly alive in at least some sense of that word. Yet the principles on which these types of biochemical exploration are based insist that if the properties of the living organism are to be understood fully, its composition and workings must continue to be explored not merely at the cellular level but at even simpler levels of organisation. Cells contain their own internal component structures. It is possible to break up the cells and separate their submicroscopic parts — the nucleus, which contains the genetic material, the mitochondria, responsible for providing the cells with a workable supply of energy derived from the burning of sugar, and so forth. Further, we can separate cells into the individual molecules of which they are composed: the proteins, lipids and carbohydrates (sugars), and the atoms of which the molecules themselves are built.

This pursuit of the properties of life down through layers of complexity to the very atoms themselves has been the major project of twentieth-century biology. The pursuit has been and is an enormously exciting story of research ingenuity. It has involved: the construction of machines capable of analysing not merely millionths but millionths of millionths of grams of complicated chemicals; the generation of powerful centrifugal fields of up to a million times gravity to separate small subcellular particles; the development of microscopes capable of magnifications of hundreds of thousands of times. The dexterity and ingenuity of the experimental manipulations match the scale of the machinery involved. Biology has become a 'big science'.

But you may well wonder where the life has gone in this *reductionist* pursuit from person to organ, from tissue to cell, from molecule to atom. Underlying this biological approach to life — and to medicine — is the belief that if one can understand the molecules and their interactions one will ultimately understand life itself, and its disorders. After all, if scurvy results from lack of vitamin C, pellagra from lack of vitamin B and diabetes from lack of insulin; if understanding of cellular processes allows the formulation of drugs that specifically interact with particular processes, with consequences for the whole organism, is not this approach justified? True, something is lost during reductionist analysis of this sort. Insulin will affect sugar metabolism (the burning of sugar for energy) in the intact organism, or in the isolated organ or tissue slice, but the moment the cells of the tissue are broken up and their constituents released, insulin ceases to exert an effect. Biochemistry depends on structure as well as molecular composition. None the less, such reductionism has been the dominant belief throughout the growth of twentieth century biology and of scientific medicine.

Reductionism's roots lie deep in the history of science. Take, for instance, the phrase we used above in discussing how the body used sugar; we referred to its 'burning' sugar, releasing carbon dioxide and providing usable energy. This word was not accidental. In the late eighteenth century the French chemist Lavoisier showed that the overall chemical reactions involved in the body's use of sugar were the same as those that took place when sugar was set on fire. In the 1820s the German chemist Wöhler showed that it was possible completely to synthesise a chemical hitherto only found in living organisms — urea, a major constituent of urine — from completely inorganic, non-living chemicals. The substances of which life is composed, therefore, and the chemical reactions that they undergo, are 'ordinary', if complicated. By the mid-nineteenth century, radical physiologists were claiming boldly that humans are what they eat, genius is a matter of phosphorus, and even that most complex organ of the body, the brain, 'secretes thought like the kidney secretes urine'.

It was not merely that life was — and still is — seen as the expression of complex chemical processes; the body's organs themselves could be visualised as working along mechanical principles. From at least the time in the seventeenth century when the English doctor William Harvey discovered the circulation of the blood, the heart was seen to function as a pump, and its workings could be described by more or less complex hydrodynamic equations. The kidney can be described as a filtration system, like a sewage plant, the brain as an information-processing system, like a computer, and so on. This mechanistic view of life is far removed from the explanatory systems offered in many other cultures.* As we

shall see, reductionist explanations 'work', but only within quite sharp limitations.

What we are saying is that there is a hierarchy of levels of organisation of biological material — from individual molecules to subcellular structures, cells, tissues, organs, the intact organism and groups of organisms in a given environment — at which biology can be studied. Within this hierarchy the level that one studies depends on the questions being asked. The more 'intact' the animal, the closer to the complexities of 'real life' will be the studies one can make; the more cellular or molecular the entities being studied, the more precise and refined the questions that can be answered. And this hierarchy does not cease 'at the border' of the organism, so to speak; no organism, certainly not a human, exists in isolation. It is part of an environment, which includes the physical world, the other biological organisms with which it comes into contact and, for humans, the social, cultural and historical framework within which each individual is embedded.

Scientific study of the properties of any living organism, human or non-human, demands the simplification of this complex environment, that one holds constant as many aspects of the phenomenon being studied as possible, changing just one. For instance, the same diet could be maintained, with or without the addition of lemon juice, to see if scurvy developed. Such simplifications and holdings of 'other things equal' are at the heart of the scientific method; they have resulted in its great achievements — yet they also limit its vision and explanatory power. For in the real world of human experience as opposed to the artificial, isolated world of experiment, the one sure thing is that other things 'are not equal'. The fact that everything is in flux and interconnected in complex ways remains a major limitation to reductionist methods.

Testing a biological hypothesis

Let us see how the methodology of experimentation within the biological hierarchy works in practice. Suppose one wants to test the hypothesis that a particular substance could be effective as a drug in the treatment of diabetes. One might begin at the level of the whole organism, by exploring the effect of the substance in a rat which showed the diabetic condition. Suppose one injects the substance, in repeated doses over several days, and finds that the rat's blood sugar level returns to normal. Can one be sure that this is the effect of the drug? Perhaps the sugar level would have corrected itself spontaneously? So *controls*, rats not injected with the drug, are necessary. But perhaps the act of injection itself may result in the sugar level returning to normal? So there must also be 'sham-injected' control rats, that is rats injected with a substance believed to be inert, perhaps chemically not too dissimilar to the drug itself.

___

* *Medical Knowledge: Doubt and Certainty* (U205, Book II) discusses some of these explanatory systems in a cross-cultural context.

How much of the drug is required to bring the blood sugar level back to normal? How many doses? Again, many trials with the appropriate controls are necessary. If the injection of a certain dose results in the correction of the blood sugar level, is this the only effect of the drug? Perhaps the drug is poisonous, or its long-term use will result in cancer. So one must ask: does the substance have other effects on the rat — on its body weight, its resistance to bacterial infection, its sexual or other behaviour? And what happens to the substance inside the rat? Is it chemically broken down, stored in body tissue, or excreted? At this stage one is likely to be moving down the hierarchy of complexity. To study the direct chemical effects of the drug on the tissue, one could use slices of liver or muscle tissue from the rat. If it works chemically (as many drugs do) by interfering with a single chemical reaction inside the cell the interaction of the new substance with isolated chemicals from the cell could be studied.

All such studies produce information of basic biological interest, and ideally, the knowledge produced by this hierarchical approach is put together to present a model of just how the substance, the proposed new drug, interacts at the molecular level with chemical processes going on inside the rat's body cells to maintain sugar metabolism at the correct level. But how relevant is this information to understanding the biology of human disease and helping to cure it? Before the drug could be introduced in therapy, it would have to be taken from the stage of known effectiveness in animals to known therapeutic value and safety in humans — the methodology of the *clinical trial*, to be discussed in Chapter 6.

Is such biological knowledge, at the cellular or molecular level, even necessary to find treatments or to alleviate suffering? As we pointed out earlier, many curative treatments have been developed empirically, that is by trial and error.

To achieve a dramatic decrease in mortality among the wounded soldiers of the Crimean War, Florence Nightingale was able to redesign hospitals in such a way as to diminish the chance of infection and contagion — without needing to know about the germ theory of disease. Epidemiological studies (Chapter 6) can indicate that the incidence of lung cancer would be dramatically reduced if people stopped smoking cigarettes, even though they cannot explain just how the tar and other products of cigarette smoke help to make the lung cells cancerous. The great prestige given in our society to 'molecular' or 'biological' explanations of disease as opposed to 'social' or 'environmental' explanations may overrate the power of biology; none the less no explanation of disease can be complete without the biological dimension.

Uses and limitations of animal models

By giving information about the biology of the 'normal', non-human organism, animal experiments help the understanding of the biological meaning of health, in infancy, adulthood and in old age. When it comes to understanding the biology of disease, everything depends on how good the animal model is. Diabetic dogs show many of the same symptoms as humans, and the symptoms can be alleviated in the same way. Insulin can be tested on animals with diabetes, because insulin works the same way in other mammals as in humans. However, there are no useful animal models for many types of human disorders. This is particularly true for psychiatric disorders. What constitutes a depressed or a schizophrenic laboratory animal, for instance? It is here that some of the problems of interpretation begin.

A further use of animal models in medical research, and one that has caused considerable controversy as it involves using a large number of animals, is to test for possible unwanted, dangerous or toxic effects of drugs or other proposed treatments. Many chemicals used in food, industry or agriculture — and in medicine itself — may have short-term or long-term deleterious effects, such as producing cancer or birth defects or increasing genetic risks. ('Carcinogenic', 'teratogenic' and 'mutagenic' are the technical terms for these three types of effect.) Legislation has therefore become more and more stringent about the need for adequate biological knowledge of the effects of any proposed new drug or analogous chemical. Such information can be derived only from studying the effects of varying (often quite high) concentrations of the drug on the short-term and longer-term life expectancy of experimental animals. The intention of such studies is to avoid a repetition of thalidomide-type disasters.

One standard test, the so-called LD_{50} test, involves exposing groups of laboratory animals to varying concentrations of the drug and noting the concentration at which 50 per cent of the exposed animals die. The difference between the therapeutic dose of the drug — the level at which it is normally administered to give a medically beneficial response — and the LD_{50} indicates the margin of safety for the drug.

Opponents of animal experimentation criticise the use of this test as particularly wasteful of animal lives and also point to its limitations. There may be differences in the way humans and other animals react to the drug (for instance, rats and humans react differently to penicillin); the test may not assess mutagenic or teratogenic dangers or the effects of long-term exposure to low concentrations adequately, and so forth. None the less, it produces a *sort* of measure of the safety (or otherwise) of the drug. At present, despite some claims to the contrary, there are no real alternatives to using *some* animals in testing the effects of new drugs or other substances. The LD_{50} test itself might be modified, and substitutes such as tissue culture could be used in a limited number of cases. But in the last analysis the question that has to be asked is not whether there is another way of discovering how safe these substances are, but whether we really need so many new drugs and other chemical additives at all?

Objectives for Chapter 3

When you have studied this chapter, you should be able to:

3.1 Understand and give examples of the use of the basic techniques of biomedical science: observation, hypothesis-making, and the testing of hypotheses by experimental intervention.

3.2 Summarise, giving examples, the basic methods available for studying the nature and causes of disease in individual humans, and their limitations: the analysis of body fluids and biopsies, the use of scanning and genetic techniques, post-mortem studies.

3.3 Define the term 'animal model' and describe the hierarchy of animal models available: intact organism, isolated organ, tissue slice, cell culture, separated cell components and molecules, and show their strengths and limitations in the search for a particular therapeutic intervention.

3.4 Distinguish between those biological effects that are the causes of disease and those that are its consequences.

Questions for Chapter 3

1 (*Objective 3.1*) From what you know of Banting and Best's discovery of the role of insulin in diabetes, describe (i) an observation they made, (ii) a hypothesis they constructed and (iii) the test of the hypothesis by experiment.

2 (*Objectives 3.2 and 3.4*) (a) Give examples of the use of (i) body-fluid analysis, (ii) genetic and (iii) post-mortem studies in the study of diabetes.

(b) What could such studies *not* tell you?

3 (*Objective 3.3*) (a) Describe three levels of analysis at which the biology of the action of insulin can be studied.

(b) Why is each level of analysis necessary?

4 (*Objective 3.3*) What could you *not* learn about the incidence of diabetes in the human population from the study of animal models such as dogs?

4

Dealing with data

Your study of Book II, *Medical Knowledge: Doubt and Certainty*, will have shown you that the methods used to study health and disease go far beyond those you met in Chapters 2 and 3 of this book. In particular, you have seen how important it is to take account of human history, rather than concentrating on individuals. The rest of this book is largely concerned with methods of studying health and disease in human societies. The methods you will meet are divided into two categories. Chapters 5 and 6 deal mainly with epidemiology, the study of the distribution of health and illness in human populations. Chapters 7–10 are concerned largely with the methods of the social sciences — ways of studying and interpreting human societies and the relationships and interactions of the people in them. As a preliminary, Chapter 4 covers some basic ideas of dealing with numerical data, which will be needed in the rest of the book and in the course. (Note that you do not have to memorise the data.)

Some of you who have more experience of dealing with numbers may find you can achieve the objectives of this chapter without working through all the detailed examples: nevertheless, we suggest you read straight through the material, doing the various activities as you come to them.

If you happen to have an electronic calculator (a very simple one will do), it would be useful to have it by you as you work through the chapter.

Everyone has been faced with the problem of dealing with numerical data. It is not easy to survive in our society without some skill at dealing with numbers, and even hard-bitten statisticians have been known to blanch at the prospect of extracting the right numbers to enter on an income tax return from a pile of crumpled papers in the bottom of a drawer. At any level, and in any context, dealing with numerical data amounts to looking for *patterns* in them — looking at how all the numbers are related to each other.

Here are some numerical data. If you have children, you will be concerned about their physical development. Are they growing properly? You might have done what many parents do — measured their height at regular intervals.

Table 4.1 Julie's height

Age/years	Height/cm
2	81
3	87
4	93
5	96

This table gives the height of a girl on four of her birthdays. When she was two, she was 81 cm (about 2 ft 8 in) tall; by the time she was five, she has grown to 96 cm (about 3 ft 2 in).

□ Can you see any patterns in these data?

■ One obvious pattern is that the older Julie gets, the taller she gets. This probably struck you as too obvious to mention! At another level, you may have noticed that she put on 6 cm in height between her second and third birthdays, and another 6 cm between her third and fourth birthdays, but only 3 cm between her fourth and fifth. That is, her growth seems to have slowed down.

This pattern might be important to Julie and her parents; does she need medical treatment?

This answer indicates that the *kind* of pattern you might look for in data depends on the kind of questions you want to ask. Julie's parents want to know if she is growing properly — so they look at the data to see how fast she is growing.

Finding patterns in data is not always as straightforward as in Julie's case: usually, the data have to be put into a form where the pattern is easier to see, and this may involve drawing a diagram like Figure 4.1, for example. This kind of diagram is called a graph. In Figure 4.1 the slowing in Julie's growth is more obvious than it was in the original table. The pattern can be made yet more obvious if the graph in Figure 4.1 is redrawn as in Figure 4.2. The

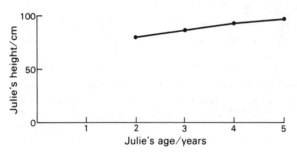

Figure 4.1 Julie's age and height.

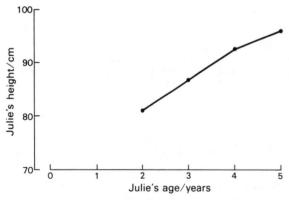

Figure 4.2 Julie's age and height shown with the height scale shortened.

scale of height, going up the side of the graph starts at 70 cm instead of zero to get rid of a lot of blank paper and make the slowing down in growth easier to see. However, a quick, uncritical glance at Figure 4.2 might give the impression that Julie's height had more than doubled between the ages of two and five, which of course is wrong. So diagrams can clarify patterns — but they can mislead!

Births — tables and histograms

You may know that one factor in determining the kind of maternity care a mother-to-be will receive is her age. The importance of the mother's age to the health of mother and child is not a simple matter. Obstetricians generally consider that women who are expecting their first child at a relatively late age are subject to a relatively high risk of things going wrong during birth. Mothers who are particularly young may be considered to be at high risk as well. Therefore, people who are concerned with planning the provision of maternity care may well need to take into account the age of mothers in their area. Let us look at some data on the age of mothers, and develop ways of presenting the data that make any underlying patterns easier to see.

Here is an example of the type of issue that can be investigated. Are Scottish mothers younger than English and Welsh mothers? How might one go about answering this question? All births in the UK have, by law, to be officially registered. Among the information collected by the Registrar is the mother's age, and her usual place of residence. So, in the offices of the Registrar General for England and Wales (in London) and the Registrar General for Scotland (in Edinburgh) are huge numbers of records of birth registration, and information based on these records is regularly published by Her Majesty's Stationery Office (HMSO). These data show there were 725 024 live births in 1980 to mothers usually resident in England, Wales and Scotland.* Of these births, 656 234 were to mothers resident in England and Wales, and the remaining 68 790 were to Scottish mothers.

In terms of mother's age, the 725 024 births can be split up into 538 725 in which the mother was aged under 30, and 186 299 in which the mother was 30 years or older.

□   Can the data presented so far be used to answer our question about the age of Scottish and English mothers?
■   No, they cannot. We have not yet told you how many of the *Scottish* mothers were under 30, for instance.

However, a partial answer to the original question can be found from Table 4.2.

This table shows that, for example, there were 485 733 live births in 1980 to mothers under 30 resident in England and Wales, and there were 15 798 live births to Scottish mothers aged 30 and over. The main part of the table has two horizontal rows, corresponding to mothers under 30 and mothers 30 and over, and two vertical columns, corresponding to the two categories of the mother's country of residence. The table also includes some figures referred to as row totals and column totals. These correspond to the figures given earlier. For example, the

---

* There were actually a small number of extra births, to mothers whose age was not recorded.

first row total is 538 725. As the name indicates, this is just the total of the figures in the corresponding row of the main part of the table. That is:

$$485\,733 + 52\,992 = 538\,725.$$

But what does that mean in words? This row total is the number of births to English and Welsh mothers aged under 30, added to the number of births to Scottish mothers under 30. So it is the total number of births to mothers under 30 in England, Wales and Scotland, which was given before as 538 725. So our numbers add up correctly! In a similar way, for example, the second column total, 68 790, is the total of the two numbers above it; so it is the total number of births to Scottish mothers. Again this agrees with the figure quoted earlier.

The remaining number in the table is the 725 024 in the bottom right-hand corner. This is just the grand total number of live births to all mothers living in England, Wales and Scotland in 1980. (So you can probably see that the two row totals should add up to this grand total, and that the two column totals should also add up to it.)

Armed with all these data, it is now possible to come up with an answer to the original question. It is clearly not true that *every* Scottish mother is younger than *every* English or Welsh mother. But do Scottish mothers *tend to be* younger than their English and Welsh counterparts? Can this question be answered on the basis of Table 4.2? The table tells us that, for example, 52 992 live births took place to Scottish mothers under 30. But this figure is not much help on its own; it must be compared with something. It *is* informative to say that: 'Out of 68 790 live births to Scottish mothers in 1980, 52 992 were to mothers aged under 30.' Or, even more usefully, 52 992 can be expressed as a *percentage* of 68 790: it is

$$\frac{52\,992}{68\,790} \times 100 \text{ per cent,}$$

that is, 77.03 per cent of 68 790. So, 'Out of 68 790 live births to Scottish mothers in 1980, 77.03 per cent were to mothers aged under 30.'

☐ Fill in the blank in this sentence: 'Out of 656 234 live births to English and Welsh mothers in 1980, _____ per cent were to mothers aged *30 or over*.' (If you have not got a calculator handy, just write down the calculations you would have to do.)

■ The required percentage is

$$\frac{170\,501}{656\,234} \times 100,$$

which comes to 25.98 per cent.

Table 4.2 is an example of a *contingency* table, which is the technical term for a table of *counts*. Each of the numbers in the table is obtained by *counting* how many mothers fall into a certain category. (Tables like this are sometimes called *cross-tabulations*.) But to answer our question, it is probably more useful to present a table of percentages, like Table 4.3.

The two percentages just calculated appear in this table: check that you understand why they appear where they do. The figures in the row marked total numbers (= 100 %) are the column totals from Table 4.2; they give the number of births to mothers from England and Wales and mothers from Scotland respectively.

☐ Express in words what the 74.02 at the top left of Table 4.3 means.

Table 4.2 Live births in 1980

Mother's age when child was born	Mother's country of residence		Row totals
	England and Wales	Scotland	
under 30	485 733	52 992	538 725
30 and over	170 501	15 798	186 299
column totals	656 234	68 790	725 024

(data from Registrar General Scotland, 1982, Table S2.6 and OPCS, 1982a, Table 7.1)

Table 4.3 Percentages of live births in 1980

Mother's age when child was born	Mother's country of residence	
	England and Wales	Scotland
under 30	74.02	77.03
30 and over	25.98	22.97
total numbers (= 100 %)	656 234	68 790

■ 'Out of the 656 234 live births to mothers living in England and Wales in 1980, 74.02 per cent were to mothers aged under 30.'

□ On the basis of these 1980 data, did Scottish mothers tend to be younger than English and Welsh mothers in that year?

■ It would appear so. Whereas the majority of mothers in all these countries was under 30, a slightly greater percentage of Scottish mothers (77 per cent) was under 30 than the corresponding percentage (74 per cent) of English and Welsh mothers.

The data in Table 4.3 can be represented in a graphical form using *pie charts* (Figure 4.3). The two 'pies' are divided up into a slice for mothers under 30 and a much smaller slice for older mothers. The size of each slice represents the number of births in the corresponding group. The English and Welsh pie is much larger than the Scottish to show there were, in total, many more births in England and Wales — in fact, the area of each pie is proportional to the number of births in the corresponding country. Again, it can be seen that a slightly greater percentage of Scottish than of English and Welsh mothers was under 30 in 1980.

Does this answer the original question? One major problem is that we have looked only at 1980 data. Other years may be different. Perhaps the 1980 age difference was just a chance fluctuation in the usual state of things. Another problem is that the age classification used was fairly rough and ready. Although a greater proportion of the Scottish mothers was aged under 30, it might be the case that most of these were *just* under 30, whereas the English and Welsh mothers aged under 30 were much younger. This possibility sounds unlikely, on the face of it; but it can be investigated by splitting up the total number of births into a larger number of mother's age categories (Table 4.4).

The column totals are the same as in Table 4.2 because both tables refer to the same births. The row totals have been omitted because we are not going to use them here. Again a table of percentages can be calculated from this contingency table (Table 4.5).

□ Does this table support the tentative conclusion that Scottish mothers tend to be younger than their English and Welsh counterparts?

■ Yes it does. In the two youngest age groups, 10.50 per cent of Scottish mothers were aged below 20, compared with only 9.26 per cent of English and Welsh, and again a higher proportion of Scottish mothers were aged between 20 and 24. A higher proportion of English and Welsh mothers fell into the older age groups.

This process of calculating a percentage table from a contingency table can be extremely useful in investigating patterns in the data in the table. In our examples, the percentages calculated have been percentages of the *column* totals; in other circumstances it·may be more useful to calculate percentages of the row totals. Often you will find that the work of calculating percentages has been done for you in published statistics. But when this has been done, be

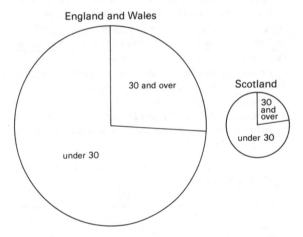

Figure 4.3 Live births in 1980, grouped according to the mother's age and country of residence.

Table 4.4 Live births in 1980

Mother's age when child was born	Mother's country of residence	
	England and Wales	Scotland
under 20	60 754	7 226
20–24	201 541	22 565
25–29	223 438	23 201
30–34	129 908	12 111
35–39	33 893	3 104
40 and over	6 700	583
column totals	656 234	68 790

(data from Registrar General Scotland, 1982, Table S2.6 and OPCS, 1982a, Table 7.1)

Table 4.5 Percentages of live births in 1980

Mother's age when child was born	Mother's country of residence	
	England and Wales	Scotland
under 20	9.26	10.50
20–24	30.71	32.80
25–29	34.05	33.73
30–34	19.80	17.61
35–39	5.16	4.51
40 and over	1.02	0.85
total numbers (= 100 %)	656 234	68 790

sure you know whether percentages of row totals or of column totals have been calculated. There is no logical or arithmetical difference between the process of calculating these two percentages — which one is calculated in a particular context depends on what the rows and columns represent *in that context*.

But even after a table of percentages has been calculated, as in Table 4.5, it can still be tricky to see the pattern in the data. The fact that Scottish mothers tend to be younger does not exactly leap out at you from the table. Often the pattern can be clearer if a diagram is drawn. Figure 4.4 shows the same information as Table 4.5, in the form of two *histograms*. Look at the England and Wales histogram first. It has six bars of equal width, each corresponding to one of the rows representing an age group in Table 4.5. The *area* of each bar represents the percentage of all live births to English and Welsh mothers in 1980 in which the mother's age fell within the appropriate range. (The percentages

have been marked above the bars in this example.) It is clear from the histogram that most births occurred to mothers in their twenties.

Fewer English and Welsh babies born in 1980 had mothers in their thirties, and even fewer had mothers under 20 or over 40. The histogram for births to Scottish mothers shows the same sort of pattern, though the area of the 'under 20' and '20 to 25' bars is slightly greater and the other bars slightly smaller than for England and Wales. This reflects the finding that, in 1980 at any rate, Scottish mothers tended to have their babies at slightly younger ages than English and Welsh mothers. But again it is worth emphasising that the difference in 1980 was small. To see if it represented a *general* pattern, we should need to look at what happened in other years.

Now let us look at further ways of representing data in diagrams.

Place of birth — graphs and relationships

In 1961 in England and Wales, only 67.5 per cent of births took place in a hospital or maternity home; almost all the rest occurred at the mother's home. By 1980, 98.7 per cent of English and Welsh babies were born in hospital. This is a massive change in the pattern of birth, which is after all an experience that all of us have to go through at least once. The reasons for the change are not simple; but an important part of the pressure for change undoubtedly came from certain parts of the medical profession, who claimed among other things that hospital birth is generally safer. Let us examine some data related to this claim.

Figure 4.5 shows the percentage of births in different places in England and Wales in each year between 1969 and 1980. The three categories of place of birth shown are the standard ones used in official statistics in England and Wales, and distinguish between hospitals where all mothers are cared for under the supervision of their general practitioner (GP) (usually small maternity units) and hospitals where maternity care is supervised by consultant obstetricians (doctors who specialise in maternity) —

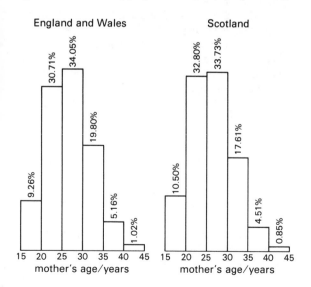

Figure 4.4 Histograms of mother's age at the time of the birth for live births in 1980.

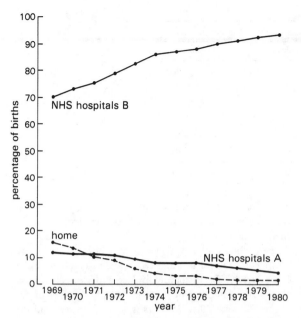

Figure 4.5 The percentage of births in England and Wales taking place in different types of establishment, 1969–80. 'NHS hospitals A' are hospitals and homes under the National Health Service (NHS) where maternity care is supervised by GPs (and not by consultant obstetricians). 'NHS hospitals B' are the remainder of hospitals and homes under the NHS (in general those with maternity care provided by consultant obstetricians). Home refers to the usual place of residence of the mother. (data from annual OPCS reports)

though these may include *some* beds where GP care is available. (The graph excludes the small numbers of births in non-NHS hospitals, and births neither at home nor in a hospital, such as births in taxis on the way to hospital.)

Look at Figure 4.5. Remember to check where the scales begin. In this instance the vertical scale starts at zero, whereas the horizontal scale of years does not.

☐ Describe the general patterns in Figure 4.5.

■ Throughout the period, most births took place in 'NHS hospitals B'. Furthermore, the proportion of births in this category rose substantially, from about 70 per cent to over 90 per cent. The proportions of births in 'NHS hospitals A' and at home both fell during the period, with home births falling more rapidly, to around 1 per cent of all births in 1980.

So, not only are fewer births taking place at home, but the births in hospital are increasingly being concentrated in (usually large) hospitals with (predominantly) consultant obstetric care rather than in (generally smaller) hospitals and maternity homes whose maternity care is supervised by general practitioners. (This is partly because fewer births were supervised by GPs and partly because GP maternity

care has largely been centralised in hospitals which have consultant obstetricians too.)

These trends are easy to see in Figure 4.5; but more detailed information can also be obtained from such graphs.

☐ What percentage of births in England and Wales took place in 'NHS hospitals A' in 1974?

■ About 8 per cent. This can be read off the graph.

☐ In which year did the proportion of births in 'NHS hospitals A' first exceed the proportion of births at home?

■ 1971. The 'NHS hospital A' and 'home' lines on the graph cross between 1970 and 1971.

☐ Did the proportion of births in 'NHS hospitals B' rise more quickly between 1970 and 1974, or between 1976 and 1980?

■ Between 1970 and 1974. In this period, the 'NHS hospital B' line on the graph rises more steeply than it does in the period 1976–80.

The question of whether these changes in the pattern of place of birth are generally desirable is difficult and strongly contested; but as we have mentioned, one claim that has been made is that birth in hospital, and in large centralised hospitals in particular, is 'safer'. But safety is not an easy thing to measure.

Suppose you wanted to compare two drivers to see which is the safer. Think about how you might do it. One possibility would be to see which driver had had the most accidents over a period of, say, five years (assuming you were in a position to collect this information).

☐ Can you think of any difficulties with this method of measurement?

■ There are several. You might have thought of the following, for example.

1 One driver might have had more accidents just because he had driven much more. As an extreme example, one driver might be a travelling salesman and drive 25 000 miles a year. In the five years, he might have had two accidents. The other driver might have driven a mile to the pub, had a crash on the way and never driven again. Which is safer?

2 Even though one driver may be less safe than the other, both of them might have escaped accidents altogether for five years. After all, even dreadful drivers crash relatively infrequently.

3 One driver might drive much more carefully than the other, but have suffered more accidents because of other careless drivers unavoidably crashing into him.

4 Getting hold of *accurate* information might not be easy. If a driver had a small accident four and a half years ago, it might not be recorded anywhere, and the driver might have forgotten about it or be unwilling to tell you about it.

So there are problems in using accidents as a measure of safety. But other measurements of safety are problematical too. You might record the number of convictions each driver had for motoring offences; but that is as problematical as counting accidents. Or you might go out driving with the two and observe their behaviour.

☐ What problems might that involve?

■ First, your presence as an observer might cause the drivers to behave differently from their normal driving style; the very act of observing may affect what is observed. (This is important in social science, and will be discussed in Chapter 8.) Second, what would you define as bad driving behaviour? (The question of defining concepts, such as safety or social class, in a way that can be *measured* is raised again in Chapter 10.)

Measuring the safety of different places of birth is even more difficult than measuring the safety of drivers. For the present, we shall use the number of *perinatal deaths* to measure the safety of maternity services. A perinatal death is officially defined as a death occurring between the twenty-eighth week of pregnancy and one week after birth, that is including still births where the child is born dead (having survived at least 28 weeks of pregnancy).

☐ In 1980, there were 622 perinatal deaths of babies whose mothers lived in the Northern Health Region (which consists of the counties of Cleveland, Cumbria, Northumberland, Durham and Tyne and Wear). The corresponding figure for the Trent Health Region (Derbyshire, Leicestershire, Lincolnshire, Nottinghamshire and South Yorkshire) was 792. Does this mean that the maternity provision in the Northern region was safer than that in the Trent region?

■ No, for many reasons. One very important reason is that the total number of births to mothers living in the two regions has not been considered. (If you do not see why this is relevant, think of a driving school that advertises 'five passes weekly'. Would you have the same opinion of the school if you knew it entered five people each week for the test as if it entered fifty?)

There were 60 783 births (live and still) to mothers in the Trent region in 1980, and 41 536 to mothers living in the Northern region. So, all other things being equal, one would expect there to be more perinatal deaths in Trent. In comparing the numbers of perinatal deaths, one must ask the question: 'Is the *proportion* of all births that lead to perinatal deaths higher in the North or in Trent?'

To answer this kind of question, we must work out, for example, how great the number of 622 perinatal deaths in the Northern region is as a proportion of the 41 536 births that took place in that region. You could work this out as a percentage; it comes to

$$\frac{622}{41\,536} \times 100 = 1.50 \text{ per cent.}$$

That is, 1.50 per cent or (1½ in every 100), of the 41 536 births to Northern region mothers in 1980 resulted in a perinatal death. In fact, this proportion is usually not expressed as a percentage, that is so many per hundred. It is conventional to express it as so many per thousand, to make the numbers easier to handle. Because 1.50 births per hundred resulted in a perinatal death in the North, one can say that 15.0 births per thousand resulted in perinatal death. This figure of 15.0 per thousand is called the *perinatal mortality rate* for births to Northern region mothers in 1980. The perinatal mortality rate (per thousand) can therefore be worked out using the formula:

$$\text{perinatal mortality rate} \atop \text{(per thousand)} = \frac{\begin{array}{c}\text{number of} \\ \text{perinatal deaths}\end{array}}{\begin{array}{c}\text{total number of} \\ \text{live and still births}\end{array}} \times 1\,000.$$

(If you are not happy with how this formula works, check that it really gives 15.0 as the perinatal mortality rate for the North.)

☐ What is the perinatal mortality rate for births to Trent region mothers in 1980? Remember there were 60 783 births and 792 perinatal deaths. (If you have not a calculator handy, just write down the formula you would use to calculate the rate.)

■ The rate is

$$\frac{792}{60\,783} \times 1\,000,$$

which comes to 13.0 per thousand.

So, although there were *more* perinatal deaths in Trent than in the Northern region in 1980, when the number of births is taken into account and the perinatal mortality rates are calculated, Trent turns out to have a *lower* rate than the Northern region.

☐ Does this mean that maternity provision in the Trent region was more effective in bringing about safer births than that in the Northern region in 1980?

■ The answer is 'not necessarily' for many reasons. Among these are the following. First, a perinatal death is a relatively rare event (in this country at any rate). A birth can be unsafe in many ways without resulting in a still birth or a baby that dies before it is a week old. For instance, the baby may be seriously ill at birth but may still survive. Even if dangerous practices were being carried out at birth, most babies would survive. Second, it might be true that the higher perinatal mortality rate in the Northern region has nothing at all to do with maternity faciles. A baby may die for reasons unconnected with the care its mother receives; for instance, it may be born with very severe congenital defects (i.e. defects that were present before birth). The Northern region might give *safer* maternity care than Trent, but still end up with a higher perinatal mortality rate.

So, just as with the two drivers and their accidents, perinatal mortality is far from being a complete measure of the safety of maternity services. One can take into account the number of births by using a *rate* (i.e. 13 per thousand) rather than just the *number* of perinatal deaths, and this idea of using rates rather than numbers is of great importance in medical statistics. But this does not avoid all the problems. And, of course, there are other ways of measuring safety in obstetrics, each with its attendant difficulties. In the meantime, let us go ahead and use perinatal mortality rates (or PNMRs), despite all their faults.

As you may know, England is divided into fourteen health regions for administrative purposes. Each of these regions has a Regional Health Authority, responsible for strategic planning and some aspects of management of the NHS services in its region. Table 4.6 presents some data for the English health regions and for Wales.

What do these figures mean, if anything? It is not easy to say just by looking at the table. Apart from anything else, it is very hard to see whether there is any pattern in the data.

Table 4.6 Percentages of births taking place in 'NHS hospitals B' and the PNMR, for mothers residing in each English health region and in Wales, 1980

Region	Percentage of all births taking place in 'NHS hospitals B'	PNMR (per 1000)
Wales	96.0	13.3
Northern	93.8	15.0
Yorkshire	94.0	14.9
Trent	91.7	13.0
East Anglian	86.0	11.3
North West Thames	96.5	11.0
North East Thames	95.7	13.8
South East Thames	96.5	12.9
South West Thames	93.9	10.8
Wessex	89.0	11.7
Oxford	91.7	12.6
South Western	86.5	12.6
West Midlands	92.7	15.1
Mersey	97.2	13.7
North Western	95.9	15.3

(data from OPCS, 1982a and 1982b)

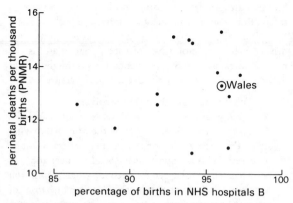

Figure 4.6 A scattergram of the percentage of births in 'NHS hospitals B' plotted against the PNMR for English health regions and for Wales in 1980.

Things are made easier if a diagram is drawn, and the appropriate kind of diagram for data such as these, in which there are *two* figures for each region, is a *scatter diagram*, or scattergram (Figure 4.6).

A scattergram starts off with two scales or *axes* (singular: axis) at right angles, like a graph. Points (small dots or crosses) are then plotted on the diagram, one for each region. We have ringed the one for Wales as an example. Notice that the scales on both axes do not start at zero. (If they did, most of the diagram would consist of blank paper!) Even on the scattergram the data do not show a clear pattern; but perhaps there is a tendency for the points on the left-hand side of the diagram to be somewhat lower than points on the right-hand side.

Other scattergrams can show clearer patterns. In Figure 4.7 each point corresponds to the height and weight of one of 30 eleven-year-old schoolgirls in Bradford. There is a clear tendency for the points to be lower on the left of diagram than on the right. But girls corresponding to points

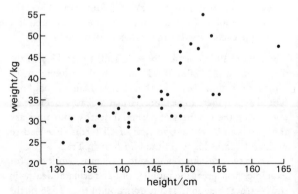

Figure 4.7 A scattergram of height and weight for 30 eleven-year-old girls. (data from Heaton Middle School, Bradford, in The Open University, 1983, Figure 3.12)

on the left are girls who are relatively short. And girls whose points are low are girls who are relatively light. So the pattern in the points merely reflects the fact that short girls tend to weigh less than tall girls. That is, the height and weight of girls are *related*. If you know a girl's height, you can make a better guess about her *weight* than you would if you knew nothing about how tall she is. Now this relationship between weight and height is not perfect. You can see from Figure 4.7 that *some* tall girls are lighter in weight than some short girls. Nevertheless, the relationship is fairly strong.

☐ Refer back to Figure 4.6. Is there a relationship between the place of birth and the PNMR data in this diagram?

■ As there is a slight tendency for the points in the figure to be lower on the left and higher on the right perhaps there is a weak relationship between the percentage of births in 'NHS hospitals B' in a health region and its PNMR.

☐ Describe what this relationship means.

■ Regions with a lower percentage of births in hospitals with consultant obstetric beds tend to have a lower PNMR. Regions with a higher percentage of births in these hospitals tend to have a higher PNMR.

☐ Does this mean that hospitals with consultant obstetric beds are more dangerous places to give birth than GP maternity units or the mother's home?

■ No. The data certainly do not disprove this, but they do not prove it either. There are many other possible explanations of the data. First, the scattergram shows only a very weak relationship. If a few of the points on it were moved a short distance, the relationship would disappear. It might be that there is no real relationship to explain. Perinatal mortality varies from one year to another anyway — perhaps the slight pattern in Figure 4.6 would not be there in another year. But even if the pattern is merely the result of a small variation from year to year, there are still other explanations. Perhaps some regions have a high PNMR because they have a lot of mothers who are very young, or very old, or at high risk in some other way. Perhaps these high-risk regions have increased the proportion of hospital births to try to *reduce* the PNMR — so in these regions the PNMR is high, but not as high as it might have been with fewer hospital births. On the other hand, it may be that consultant obstetric beds do increase the PNMR. The point is that *you cannot tell from these data alone.*

Whenever a relationship between two quantities is found in data, great care must be taken in interpreting it. You *cannot* infer that the *relationship* is *causal*, that changes in one of the quantities cause changes in the other. (At least, you cannot make this inference from the data alone; other

things must be taken into account. We shall return to this point in Chapter 6.)

So the data in Table 4.6 and Figure 4.6 did not tell us much. There was only a weak relationship between the PNMR and the place of birth, and even if it had been strong it would not have meant that hospital consultant care necessarily raised the PNMR — or lowered it for that matter. But before leaving this subject, it is worth looking at a few more data. The data in Table 4.6 were *cross-sectional*; that is, the table gave figures for a lot of different places at one point in time. Another possibility is to look at *longitudinal* data — data for *one* place at *many* points in time. In Figure 4.8 each point corresponds to the percentage of births in 'NHS hospitals B' and the PNMR for the same place — actually the whole of England and Wales, but for eleven different years, 1970 to 1980. Each point has a label showing which year it corresponds to.

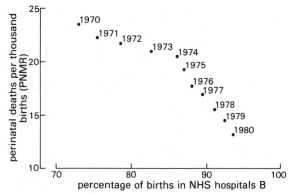

Figure 4.8 A scattergram of the percentage of births in 'NHS hospitals B' plotted against the PNMR for England and Wales, 1970–80. (data from annual OPCS reports)

This scattergram shows a very clear pattern, but the points go the opposite way to those in Figure 4.6. In Figure 4.8 the points are high up on the left and low down on the right; they slope down from left to right. If the scattergram looks like this, the two quantities involved are said to have a *negative relationship*. In Figures 4.6 and 4.7 the points tended to slope upwards from left to right. When this happens the two quantities are said to have a *positive relationship*. (Note that here the words 'positive' and 'negative' are being used in a purely mathematical sense — they have no evaluative connotations.) You should be aware that some relationships are neither positive nor negative, as in Figure 4.9 (overleaf).

The negative relationship in Figure 4.8 says that, between 1970 and 1980, the greater the proportion of births in consultant obstetric units was, the lower the PNMR became. Now this observation has been used to support the argument that obstetric units are safer.

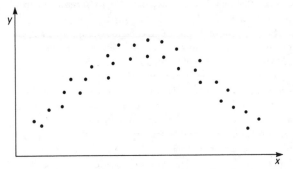

Figure 4.9 A scattergram showing a relationship that is neither positive nor negative.

☐ Does it *prove* that consultant obstetric units are safer?

■ No. The pattern in the data is rather too strong to admit the possibility that it is simply the result of random variation. But apart from all the problems of whether the PNMR is a good measure of safety, there is nothing in these data to show that increasing the proportion of births in 'NHS hospital B' *caused* the PNMR to fall. This might be so, but it might also be that some other factor caused the PNMR to fall coincident-ally with the rise in obstetric unit births. It might even be that the PNMR would have fallen *faster* if the rise in obstetric unit births had not occurred.

Perhaps the main thing to learn from Figures 4.6 and 4.8 is that there appears to be a positive relationship in the cross-sectional data (Figure 4.6) and a negative relationship in the longitudinal data (Figure 4.8). This does not always occur. In Figure 4.7 the data were cross-sectional in that they referred to a lot of different people all measured at the same time, and for these people the relationship between height and weight is positive. But if you measured the height and weight of an individual child growing up through the years, the child would be light and short when she was young, and heavy and tall when she was older. That is, her height and weight would still have a positive relationship in these longitudinal data. The point here is that you *cannot tell* what a relationship in longitudinal data will be like by looking at cross-sectional data (and vice versa).

Well, where have we got to? As a student, you should have learned something about dealing with and interpret-ing data in graphs and scattergrams. But what about the question we were investigating? Originally, this question was whether consultant obstetric units were safer places to be born in. But there were problems in measuring safety and, even ignoring these, the data we looked at were certainly not conclusive. In a sense they seemed to be contradictory, with a positive cross-sectional relationship and a negative longitudinal one. So an answer to the original question is still a long way off. Perhaps you will be consoled by the observation that interesting questions hardly ever have easy answers; often, that is just what makes them interesting!

Gestation — averages and variability

How long does human pregnancy last? Well, everyone must know that a figure of 9 months comes into the picture somewhere. You have probably read, or been told, at some time that the average length of human pregnancy (or the length of gestation, to use the biological term) is about 40 weeks, measured from the start of the mother's last menstrual period. Some babies are born prematurely. Others are born late. What status does the 40 weeks figure have? It is an average, but what does that mean? To help you to learn more about what an average is, and what it can and cannot tell you, let us look at some data.

Ten pregnancies lasted the following numbers of weeks: 40, 43, 36, 43, 33, 30, 41, 35, 41, 40. Figure 4.10 is a histogram of these data. Only two of these pregnancies lasted 40 weeks. One was as short as 30 weeks, and two lasted 43 weeks. But it is difficult to see much pattern in so few data. If you had to choose a single number to represent these 10 numbers perhaps 40 would not be a bad choice. It is somewhere in the middle of the range. In fact, as many of the numbers are less than 40 as are greater than 40, and because of this 40 is called the *median* of this set of data.

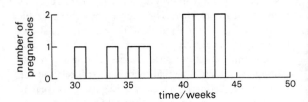

Figure 4.10 The duration of ten pregnancies.

Another very common way of finding a single number to represent a whole batch of numbers is to calculate their *mean*. This is done as follows:

1 Add up all the numbers in the batch to give their total.

2 Count how many numbers there are in the batch; that is, find the size of the batch.

3 Then,

$$\text{the mean} = \frac{\text{total}}{\text{size}}.$$

Strictly speaking, this procedure, gives you the *arithmetic mean*. This is what people are usually talking about then they refer to an average. There are other types of mean, but when we use the term it is the arithmetic mean we are after.

The mean of the data on length of pregnancies can be found as follows:

1 Total = 40 + 43 + 36 + 43 + 33 + 30 + 41 + 35 + 40 + 41, which comes to 382.

2 Size = 10 because there are 10 numbers in the batch.

3 So,

$$\text{the mean} = \frac{\text{total}}{\text{size}} = \frac{382}{10} = 38.2.$$

That is, the mean of the lengths of gestation is 38.2 weeks — rather less than 40 weeks.

But one cannot tell much from only 10 pregnancies. Figure 4.11 is a histogram of the length of gestation of

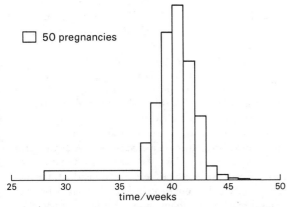

Figure 4.11 The duration of pregnancies of 2 803 women at the Royal Women's Hospital, Melbourne, 1965–67. (data from Beischer *et al.*, 1969, pp.479 and 481)

almost 3 000 pregnancies, which occurred in Australia in 1965–67. In this histogram, the bars are not all of equal width. For example, a single bar represents all pregnancies lasting between 28 and 37 weeks (because the exact lengths of those pregnancies were not given in the original data). But its *area* still represents the number of pregnancies lasting between 28 and 37 weeks.

☐ How would you describe the pattern in Figure 4.11?

■ Most of the pregnancies lasted somewhere round 40 weeks — and 40 weeks was in fact the most common length of gestation. (Because of this, 40 weeks is called the *mode* of this set of data.) But a few of the pregnancies lasted much longer or shorter times than this. Some lasted only 28 weeks; others lasted well over 40 weeks. One actually lasted 47 weeks.

The mean duration of gestation for the 2 803 pregnancies in Figure 4.11 was 39.6 weeks. Looking at the histogram, it seems that this figure represents the lengths of gestation pictured there as well as any single figure could. But finding the mean of this set of data is not the only way to find a single representative figure. Two other ways which have been mentioned briefly are to find the mode or the median. The mode is simply the most common value; so we have stated the mode of the data in Figure 4.11 is 40 weeks. The median of a set of numbers is the middle value when the numbers are arranged in order. So it turns out that the median duration of gestation of all the pregnancies in Figure 4.11 is 40 weeks as well.

You might be wondering why anyone bothers with all three of the mean, median and mode — for the data in Figure 4.11 they all come out to be about the same. But this does not always happen. Look at Figure 4.12, which shows the gross weekly earnings of a sample of over 81 000 male employees in Britain for one week in April 1980. The mean and the median are marked on the histogram, and they

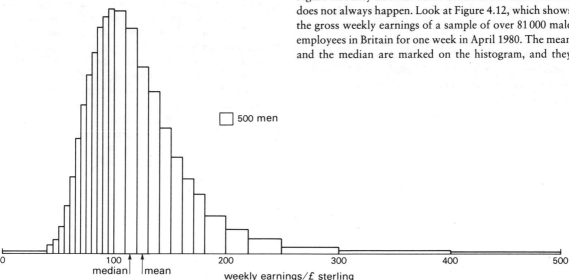

Figure 4.12 The gross weekly earnings for one week in April 1980 of a sample of 81 352 British men aged over 21. (data from Department of Employment, 1980, Table 19)

differ quite considerably. The median is £113.30 because exactly half of the men in question earned less than £113.30, and the rest earned more. So £113.30 is a reasonably representative figure for the level of earnings of these men. The mean, however, is rather larger than this. Over 60 per cent of these men earned less than the mean.

☐ Can you explain why the mean is greater than the median in this case? (Think about the way the mean is calculated, and about the general shape of the histogram in Figure 4.12.)

■ Looking at Figure 4.12, you can see that the histogram is spread out much more thinly on the right-hand side than on the left. This reflects the fact that there are a few men (to the far right of the histogram) who earn far more than the general level of earnings. The mean is calculated by adding up the gross earnings of the 81 352 men, and dividing this total by 81 352. So it is the amount each man would get if they lumped all their earnings together and divided the total up equally. The large amounts earned by a few have the consequence that far more of the men would receive higher earnings than would receive less if this sharing were done. The median is much less affected by these few people with atypically high incomes.

So the median and mean both represent the general level of earnings, but they do so in different ways. Which is most appropriate depends on the question being considered. In other circumstances, the mean can be less than the median, and the mode is very often different from both. All three are types of average, in that each is a single figure that represents the general level of a set of figures. But one figure very rarely tells the whole story.

Figure 4.13 is a histogram of the length of gestation of 819 pregnancies in cows. The mean length of gestation here is 40.5 weeks, very close to the mean length of human gestation. Yet the pattern in Figure 4.13 is very different from that in Figure 4.11.

☐ What is the main difference?

■ The *spread* of the lengths of gestation in Figure 4.13 is much less than that in Figure 4.11.

You may be able to think of reasons why this should be so. But whether there is a reason for the difference or not, Figures 4.11 and 4.13 demonstrate that there is more to a set of figures than just their mean.

In the short-term planning of maternity services, the length of (human) gestation must be taken into account. If a maternity hospital knows well in advance when mothers are going to give birth, it can plan its services efficiently, and anticipate peaks in demand for maternity beds. Yet Figure 4.11 shows that this planning can never be perfect. Babies can arrive unexpectedly early or late. The hospital must plan on the basis that whereas most pregnancies will last about 40 weeks, a substantial proportion will be two or three weeks longer or shorter, and a few will be longer or shorter still. Maternity unit administrators might look longingly at Figure 4.13 — if they were providing a service for cows, things would be simpler. Again, not all bovine pregnancies last exactly 40 weeks, but the vast majority lasted between 39 and 41 weeks.

So the spread of a batch of data can have great importance. You may have met various ways of measuring the spread numerically (the standard deviation, the variance and the interquartile range are perhaps the most common). We shall not explain further exactly what these terms mean; but you should be aware that the more widely spread out the data are, the larger these measures of spread will be. The idea of spread plays an important part in formal statistical methods of making decisions. This will be discussed again in Chapter 6, but the general idea is as follows. Suppose one were interested in whether a particular group of women tended to have longer pregnancies than average. One would probably look at the length of gestation of pregnancies of women in the group to see whether they were unusually long. But what does 'unusually long' mean? A human pregnancy lasting 42 weeks is not really unusually long — but a cow's pregnancy lasting 42 weeks *is* probably unusual, on the evidence of Figure 4.13. What is unusual in this context depends on the spread, and so any decision on whether this particular group of women was unusual must depend on the spread of the length of pregnancy in women in general.

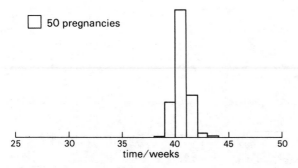

☐ 50 pregnancies

Figure 4.13 The duration of pregnancies of 819 cows (data from the Milk Marketing Board).

Objectives for Chapter 4

When you have studied this chapter, you should be able to:

4.1 Interpret data presented in contingency tables, and calculate row and column percentages where appropriate.

4.2 Describe the basic pattern of data presented in a histogram, in a graph or in a scatter diagram.

4.3 Define perinatal mortality rate.

4.4 Say what is meant by a relationship between two quantities, and distinguish between positive and negative relationships.

4.5 Distinguish between longitudinal and cross-sectional data.

4.6 Calculate the mean of a (small) batch of data, say what is meant by the median and the mode and, in general terms, by the spread of a batch of data.

Questions for Chapter 4

1 (*Objective 4.6*) The following data are the heart rates (in beats per minute) of eight patients after receiving a certain drug: 90, 82, 95, 80, 88, 75, 83, 90. What is the mean heart rate of these patients?

2 (*Objectives 4.2 and 4.3*) This question uses some data on social class, using the Registrar General's Social Classes. In this system, people are assigned to a social class according to their job. Broadly, there are five classes: I (professional), II (intermediate), III (skilled), IV (partly skilled) and V (unskilled). In the data here, the social class of a baby is defined by its father's occupation and only legitimate births are included.

(a) In 1979, there were 89 397 births (live and still) of babies whose fathers were in social class IV. Of these, 1 479 resulted in perinatal deaths. What is the perinatal mortality rate for the babies of fathers in social class IV?

(b) Figure 4.14 shows the corresponding PNMR for 1979 for all five social classes. Describe the pattern in these data.

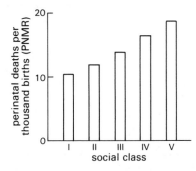

Figure 4.14 The variation in the PNMR for legitimate babies born in 1979 in England and Wales, according to the father's social class. (data from OPCS, 1982e, Table 7)

3 (*Objective 4.1*) Table 4.7 is derived from the 1981 Census, and gives the usually resident population of two neighbouring districts of Buckinghamshire, broken down according to age.

(a) Calculate the row percentages for this table.

(b) Describe the general pattern in the data shown by these percentages.

Table 4.7

District	Age group				Row total
	0–19	20–39	40–64	65 and over	
Milton Keynes	42 715	42 663	26 681	11 237	123 296
Aylesbury Vale	41 074	39 812	34 743	15 142	130 771

4 (*Objectives 4.4 and 4.5*) In this scatter diagram (Figure 4.15) each dot corresponds to a group of men who have a particular type of occupation, such as 'miners and quarrymen' or 'sales workers'. The quantity on the horizontal axis is a measure of the average amount smoked by men in the occupational group in 1972–3; the greater this figure the more they smoke.

The quantity on the vertical axis is a measure of the average death rate from lung cancer in each group in 1970–72; the greater the number, the greater the importance of lung cancer as a cause of death for that group. (The calculation of these standardised mortality ratio figures is described in Chapter 5.)

(a) These two variables are related. Is the relationship positive or negative?

(b) How would you describe the relationship in words?

(c) Does the relationship show that smoking causes lung cancer?

(d) Are these data longitudinal or cross-sectional?

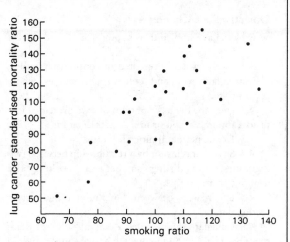

Figure 4.15 The relationship between lung cancer and smoking habits for various occupational groups of men. (redrawn from OPCS, 1978, Figure 6.3)

5

Some basic ideas of demography and epidemiology

If you have done little mathematics recently, you may find the section on birth and death rates (pp. 37–46) heavy going. If so, we suggest you read through it quickly to get the general picture, and then work through in detail. On the other hand, if you are familiar with this kind of material a quick read through may be all you need to achieve the objectives.

Again you will find an electronic calculator handy.

When Mr Lawson (whom you met in Chapter 2) visited his doctor with a health problem, he expected her to be interested in him and in his problem. He would not expect his GP to start talking about how many people in his town or his country had the same disease, where they lived and what they ate. He would probably be even more surprised if his doctor had made similar comments about people who did *not* have diabetes. Clinical medicine is traditionally centred round the patient, and other people are considered only insofar as they affect the patient. Other approaches take a broader view; they take large groups of people as the basis for study, and look at patterns of disease in whole communities, whole societies, or even the whole world.

☐ One method of clinical enquiry discussed in Chapter 2 does go further than looking at patients one at a time. Can you remember what it was?

■ The *case series*, in which a number of individuals with the same condition are observed, in a search for some factor common to them all.

The example of a case series described in Chapter 2 involved the discovery that many people suffering from nasopharyngeal cancer had been woodworkers. Yet it took further research to establish that the cancer was *caused* by materials to which the woodworkers were exposed. This research involved investigating not only woodworkers with cancer, but also other people with the same type of cancer, and indeed people who did *not* have this cancer. By the end of the next chapter, you should be able to see why this was necessary.

Approaches to studying health and disease as they occur in large groups of people may seem at first to be too depersonalised, almost inhuman somehow. Surely it is individuals who get diseases? But people do not exist in isolation from one another; we live in societies, large and small. In this chapter you will encounter some of the basic ideas and terms used in discussing health and disease at the level of substantial groups of people. These ideas come from fields of study known as demography and epidemiology.

Demography is the study of whole populations of people, with particular reference to the numbers of people involved. Demographers are interested in such matters as how many people live in a particular geographical area, how old they are, how many are female and how many male, how many are born, get married or die each year. They study how quickly these numbers change, whether they are increasing or decreasing, and forecast how they may change in the future. The basic data of demography come from censuses, registrations of births, deaths and marriages, and similar sources. The methods used by demographers have links with geography, mathematics and statistics. Demography itself is not usually seen as a branch of health studies, but its relevance to health and disease is considerable. Demographers are interested in birth and death; so are doctors. Health service planners need to know *how many* people need maternity beds or dental services. Finally, epidemiologists use demographic information as a basis for their work.

Epidemiology sounds as if it ought to mean the study of epidemics. It does include this, but the term is much wider. It describes the study of the distribution and determinants of disease in human populations. The field of study of epidemiology can be divided into three main areas, in the context of this book. They could be summarised rather crudely as: 'Who gets ill?', 'Why do they get ill?' and 'How should they be treated?'. The first area consists of the description of patterns of disease in populations, and involves the measurement of mortality, morbidity (illness) and disability. It is in this area that epidemiology and demography have most in common. You have already seen a brief example of this kind of work in the discussion of PNMR in the last chapter; in the rest of this chapter we shall concentrate on the methods used to study these topics.*

The second area of epidemiology we shall consider is the *aetiology* of disease; that is, the study of what causes disease. A famous example of an epidemiological study in this area was John Snow's work on cholera. Snow (1813–58) was interested in the role of drinking water in the spread of cholera. In studying the 1848 London cholera epidemic he found that people who had drunk water provided by a particular water company were much more likely to contract the disease than those who had not. The

company in question drew its water from the Thames near a point where vast quantities of sewage were discharged. This supported the hypothesis that the disease was transmitted by something carried in drinking water as opposed to hypotheses involving direct transmission between individuals, or miasma, which were current at the time. (Snow was working before the theory of infection by germs or microbes had been established.) In 1854 there was another major cholera outbreak in London. Snow noted the location of all the cholera cases in Soho, and later plotted them on a map. He found that all these people had drunk water from a pump in Broad Street (now called Broadwick Street). People using nearby wells had escaped the disease. Snow managed to get the handle of the Broad Street pump removed, and the outbreak stopped (though, to spoil the story rather, it has been claimed that the outbreak was coming to a halt anyway).

Although doubtless Snow was *concerned* about the individuals in Soho, his study did not concentrate on them *as individuals*. He was interested in the patterns of where the victims lived and where they got their water, and of where the people who escaped the disease got *their* water. Yet his study led directly to a better understanding of the disease at the individual level, and ultimately to the control of the disease in Western countries.

Snow's work brings out two important points about epidemiology. First, epidemiology is a science. It aims to describe and explain things in the natural world. It is a science that operates at the level of populations. But its findings can be applied to individuals. Snow's work on cholera contributed to the survival of many individuals who might otherwise have died of the disease. Second, because epidemiology works at the population level, it cannot directly provide explanations in terms of what happens within the individual. Snow found that drinking certain water caused cholera. The link between drinking water contaminated by sewage and cholera was established long before it was known exactly what it was about the contaminated water that caused cholera, or how it acted in the sufferer's body to produce symptoms of the disease. To study such causes, biological methods are needed.

The third area of epidemiology discussed here is the study of what happens after a person has a disease. Epidemiological methods can be used to investigate the effectiveness of a treatment for a disease, and of the health service that provides the treatment. How many people does it cure? Is a new treatment better than an existing one? Is prevention better than cure? Is Mr Lawson's diabetes likely to shorten his life? How should the health service be organised to cope with people like Mr Lawson? Methods for evaluating treatments are dealt with in Chapter 6; but before studying such matters we must begin with counting births and deaths.

---

* *The Health of Nations* (U205, Book III) is also largely concerned with this area of study.

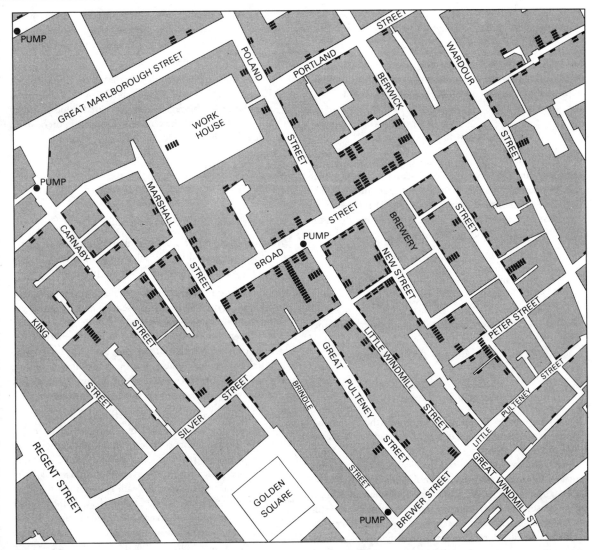

Figure 5.1 A portion of Snow's map of the spread of cholera in Soho. Bars represent the number of fatal cases in each house. The position of the Broad Street pump from which all the victims had obtained water is also marked.

Counting and comparing births and deaths

How do demographers count births and deaths? And how do they compare numbers of births and deaths at different places and at different times? In the last chapter we stated that 656 234 births occurred in 1980 to mothers resident in England and Wales, and that this figure was calculated on the basis of registration returns. (A national system of registration of births and deaths (and marriages) has been in operation in England and Wales since 1837, though the practice of registering christenings, burials and weddings in parish registers had been going on since the sixteenth century.)

□ In 1930, there were 648 811 births to English and Welsh mothers. Does this mean that the English and Welsh population was more fertile in 1980 than in 1930?

■ It all depends what is meant by 'more fertile'. In one sense, the 1980 population was more fertile because it produced more babies. But in 1980 there were an estimated 49 244 300 people living in England and Wales, compared with only about 39 800 000 in 1930.*

---

* Unless otherwise stated, figures for British births, deaths and populations in this chapter are taken from official OPCS publications (particularly OPCS 1981, 1982a, 1982c and 1982d).

So, just as with perinatal deaths, if we are to compare like with like, in comparing the births in 1980 and 1930, we must look at *birth rates*.

For 1980, 656 234 babies were born from a population of 49 244 300. The birth rate (per cent) is the number of births expressed as a percentage of the population; that is,

$$\frac{656\,234}{49\,244\,300} \times 1000$$

which comes to 1.33 per cent. As with the perinatal mortality rate (PNMR), it is more usual to express birth rates per thousand rather than per cent (per hundred). The birth rate per thousand is then ten times the birth rate per cent, that is 13.3 per thousand. The birth rate per thousand can be found directly using this formula:

$$\begin{matrix} \text{(crude) birth rate} \\ \text{per thousand in a} \\ \text{particular year} \end{matrix} = \frac{\begin{matrix} \text{number of} \\ \text{births that year} \end{matrix}}{\begin{matrix} \text{total population} \\ \text{that year} \end{matrix}} \times 1000.$$

(This rate is called the crude rate in comparison with other types of rate you will meet later.)

For 1930, the crude birth rate per thousand was

$$\frac{648\,811}{39\,800\,000} \times 1000$$

which comes to 16.3. You could interpret this by saying, 'For every thousand people living in England and Wales in 1930, 16.3 babies were born'.

But you have just read that in *1980*, 13.3 babies were born per thousand people living in England and Wales. So although *more* babies were born in 1980 than in 1930, it seems reasonable to say that the population was *less* fertile in 1980 than in 1930 because the birth rate was lower.

Birth rates, death rates, and various other kinds of rates, are widely used in demography and epidemiology. They enable comparisons to be made between numbers of births, for example, at different times and places, taking account of the size of the population involved. Using a birth rate, one can check whether an increase in *numbers* of births is merely caused by an increase in the size of the population. But this can be done only if more information is available. Births are actually counted as they occur, by the Registrars' Offices. However, to calculate birth rates, the size of the population is needed as well, and the population is counted only once every ten years, at the census. So birth rates for years between censuses have to be based on *estimates* of the population, and because of that they may be less accurate than figures for total numbers of births. This inaccuracy will probably be negligible when birth rates for the whole country are calculated, but can be more of a problem in

birth rates for smaller areas. (In Third World countries, where birth registration may be patchy or non-existent and censuses rare and inaccurate, it is much more difficult to estimate the birth rate.)

☐ In the last chapter you saw that in the Trent Health Region, there were 60 783 live births in 1980. The total population of the region was estimated to be 4 555 200 in 1980. What was the crude birth rate? (If you have no calculator, just write down the calculation you would do.)

■ The rate is

$$\frac{60\,783}{4\,555\,200} \times 100$$

which comes to 13.3 per thousand.

Although it is very useful to compare numbers of births with the total population, by calculating a crude birth rate, it is not always the most useful way to proceed.

☐ Can you think of some problems that might arise when the crude birth rate is used? (Think about where the babies actually come from!)

■ There are several problems, but perhaps the most important is that the *total* population includes a large number of people who cannot give birth: men, young girls and women over childbearing age. This might distort the picture given by the crude birth rate.

One area might have a low crude birth rate, not because its women are not very fertile, but because there is an unusually large proportion of men in its population. The number of births per thousand people would be low, therefore, only because most of every thousand people were men. To avoid presenting a misleading picture, it might be necessary to compare the number of births with the number of women in the population capable of giving birth. To do this, one would need to know how many such women there were — not an easy thing to estimate. But what *can* be done is to use an estimate of the number of women of childbearing age, and this is very often taken as being the number of women aged 15 to 44 inclusive. This figure is used to calculate what is known as the general fertility rate:

$$\begin{matrix} \text{general fertility rate} \\ \text{(per thousand)} \end{matrix} = \frac{\text{number of births}}{\begin{matrix} \text{number of women} \\ \text{aged 15–44} \end{matrix}} \times 1000.$$

In England and Wales in 1980, there were estimated to be 10 094 900 women aged 15–44, so the general fertility rate was

$$\frac{656\,234}{10\,094\,900} \times 1000 = 65.0 \text{ per thousand.}$$

That is, for every thousand women of childbearing age, 65 gave birth that year.

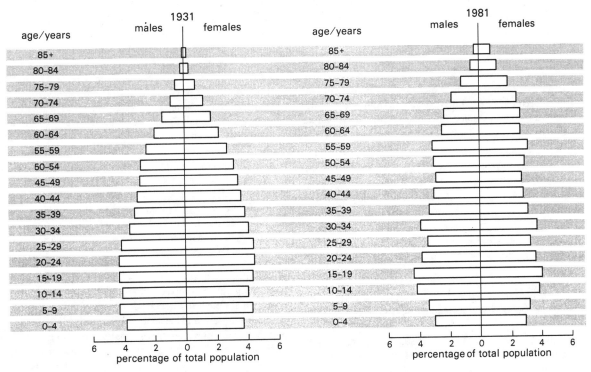

Figure 5.2 Population pyramids for England and Wales in 1931 and 1981. (data from official census reports)

□ Thus, in 1980 for England and Wales the crude birth rate was 13.3 per thousand and the general fertility rate was 65.0 per thousand. In 1932, the crude birth rate was higher, at 15.3 per thousand, but the general fertility rate was lower at 62.6 per thousand. Can you think of any reasons why this might be so? (Think about the number of old people in the population in 1932, compared with the number of young women.)

■ It was because women of childbearing age made up a greater proportion of the total population in 1932 than in 1980. In 1932 women aged 15–44 accounted for about 25 per cent of the total population: the corresponding figure for 1980 was around 21 per cent. The crude birth rate was lower in 1980 than in 1932, largely because the population included a lower proportion of young women (and many more old people).

Thus, to understand fertility within a population, it may be necessary to look beyond the total size of the population and to consider the *population structure*, that is the age and sex of the people. But for this, more information is needed. (Age and sex are recorded at the census, but for years between censuses, detailed estimates have to be made.)

One method of picturing the way a population is broken up into groups according to age and sex is the *population pyramid*. Figure 5.2 shows population pyramids for the populations of England and Wales at the censuses of 1931 and 1981. The length of each bar represents the proportion of the total population that is in that particular age–sex group. Thus the bottom left-hand bar on the 1931 pyramid indicates that, at the 1931 census, 3.8 per cent of the total population consisted of males aged 0–4 years.

□ What would you say were the most obvious differences between the age and sex structures of the populations in England and Wales in 1931 and 1981? (Look at the differences in shape between the two pyramids in Figure 5.2, and work out what they mean in terms of the populations.)

■ Perhaps the most noticeable feature is that the 1981 diagram is wider at the top, which means that a greater proportion of people were old, as we have mentioned. The bars corresponding to women aged 15–44 are longer in the 1931 pyramid than in the 1981 pyramid, again confirming what has been said before. Two other notable features in the 1981 pyramid are the 'waist', showing that there were relatively few people aged between about 40 and 50 in that year, and the fact that there were far more women than men in the older age groups.

☐ In what years were the people aged 40–50 in 1981 born? Can you think why there are relatively few of them?

■ They must have been born between 1931 and 1941. There are two possible reasons why they are few in number. Either relatively few of them were born in the first place, or more of them died before 1981 than might have been expected. The first explanation is the more relevant in this instance; birth rates in the 1930s and in the first part of the 1939–45 World War were low.

But the explanation for the preponderance of older women over older men cannot be explained in terms of births, so let us leave births for the time being, and turn our attention to the other end of the life cycle. Deaths interest demographers just as much as births, and they can be studied using similar tools. Numbers of deaths are collected through the registration process. They can be used to calculate the crude death rate, using the formula:

$$\text{crude death rate (per thousand) in a particular year} = \frac{\text{number of deaths that year}}{\text{total population that year}} \times 1\,000.$$

So for England and Wales in 1980, there were 581 385 deaths out of a population of 49 244 300, giving a crude death rate of

$$\frac{581\,385}{49\,244\,300} \times 1\,000$$

which comes to 11.8 per thousand. That is, out of every thousand people in England and Wales in 1980, 11.8 of them died (on average).

However, you may well suspect from the discussion of the crude birth rate that there can be difficulties in using the crude death rate. In England and Wales in 1976, the crude death rate was 12.1 per thousand. The corresponding death rate for Mexico in the same year was only 7.3. Does this surprise you? Surely Mexico is a rather poor country, with health services less developed than those in England and Wales?

☐ Can you think of an explanation for this apparent paradox?

■ The discussion of the birth rate may have led you to suspect that the age and sex structures of the populations are involved. They are!

With birth rates, it made sense to calculate the general fertility rate, which ignores men, and women outside the childbearing years. Now, everyone can die, but not everyone has the same chance of dying in a given year. An 82-year-old man is more likely to die in the year than, say, a 26-year-old woman. Figure 5.3 shows the population pyramids for Mexico and for England and Wales in 1976.

☐ How do they differ?

■ The England and Wales pyramid is, not surprisingly, very similar in shape to the 1981 pyramid in Figure 5.2. But the Mexico pyramid is a completely different shape. It really *is* a pyramid, with a vast preponderance of children and young people. (The is largely because birth rates are very high, and the total size of the population is growing rapidly. The fact that death rates are relatively high as well also contributes to this type of population structure.)

☐ How does this difference in the age structures of the populations explain the difference in crude death rates?

■ A far greater proportion of the Mexican population consists of young people, who, relatively speaking, are less likely to die in a given year than old people are. So the crude death rate in Mexico will be lower than it would be if Mexico had the same population age structure as England and Wales.

How can the death rates in countries with different population age structures be compared? There are several approaches. One is to calculate death rates for different age groups separately, and because the chance of dying depends on sex as well, these *age-specific death rates* are generally calculated separately for the two sexes. (This, of course, means that the *age* of people who die must be recorded.) For example, in England and Wales in 1976 there were an estimated 1 392 400 women aged 65–69, and in that year 27 538 women aged 65–69 died. So the age-specific death rate (per thousand) for females of age 65–69 was

$$\frac{27\,538}{1\,392\,400} \times 1\,000$$

which comes to 19.8 per thousand. Figure 5.4 shows the age-specific death rates for males and for females in Mexico and England and Wales in 1976. The general shape of all four lines on the graph is the same. For both sexes and in both countries the age-specific death rate falls during childhood, and then gradually rises with age, in what is known as a 'bathtub' shape. Age-specific death rates for all countries have this characteristic shape. At all ages, in both Mexico and England and Wales, the age-specific death rates for males are above the rates for females of the same age. This is true for *most* countries, though in some less developed countries the difference is much smaller. For example, in certain areas of India, mortality rates for females are *higher* than those for males.

But, most importantly for our story, at all ages the Mexican death rates for females are well above those for England and Wales. This confirms that the lower *crude* death rate in Mexico is due to the very different age structure of the population there. At any given age, a Mexican woman is *more* likely to die than an English

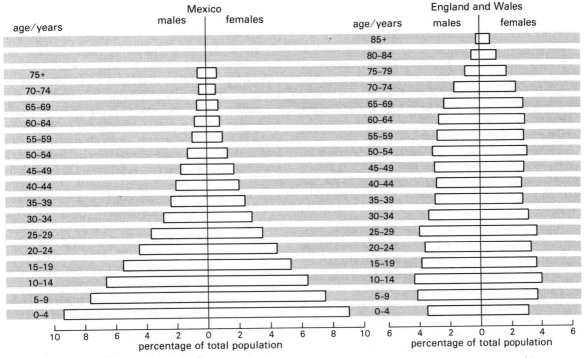

Figure 5.3 Population pyramids for Mexico and England and Wales in 1976. (data from United Nations, 1977, pp.200 and 216)

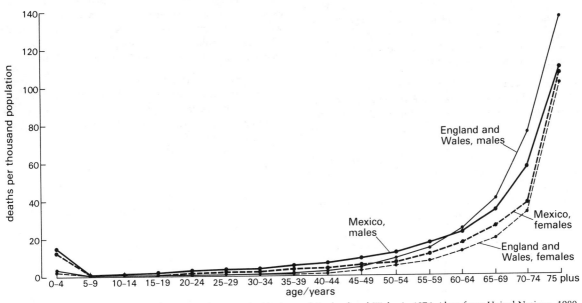

Figure 5.4 Age-specific death rates for men and women in Mexico and England and Wales in 1976. (data from United Nations, 1980, pp.580 and 604)

woman, but the difference in age structure disguises this. The picture for men is not so clear-cut.

Although the age-specific death rates provide a fairly complete picture of the mortality in an area, they have the disadvantage that they provide thirty-odd figures to work with rather than only one. So various ways have been used to compare death rates *allowing* for differences in age structure, while still using only one rate, or more usually two (one for each sex). First let us look at one of these methods, which involves calculating what is called the *expectation of life* or *life expectancy*.

Life expectancy is, roughly speaking, a measure of average length of life. The basic idea behind it is that in places with high mortality, *on average* people do not live very long. However, life expectancy is not just the mean length of life of an actual group of people.

□ Can you see why this is so? (Think about *which* group of people you would have to find the mean length of life for, to give a measure of the mortality in Mexico in 1976. Remember we are trying to avoid distortions produced by the age structure.)

■ The main problems arise because population size, age structure, and age-specific death rates change over time. Suppose the mean length of life of all those who died in Mexico in 1976 were calculated. The population contains a preponderance of young people, and one would be amalgamating deaths of these young people with deaths of old people, born many years before, when the whole population was smaller. So the average length of life of those who died in 1976 would come out to be *less* than it would be if the Mexican age structure were more like that of England — even if the age-specific death rates were the same. So this method does not allow for age structure.

Another approach would be to look at the average length of life of all the people *born* in the same year, a so-called *birth cohort* of people. This would avoid the problem of age structure, because at any time all these people are the same age. But which birth year should be taken? The year 1976 is no good, because the average could not be calculated until all the 1976 babies had eventually died, in 100 years time or so. And choosing some year in the past would not do either. Suppose the cohort born in 1876 were chosen. Almost all of them would have died by 1976, so assuming the data could be collected (which it probably could not), their average age at death could be found. But this would not tell you much about mortality *in 1976*. The problem is that people live through time, and any kind of average length of life will be affected by death rates in many different years.

Life expectancy, therefore, is calculated not from the average lifetimes of *real* people, but from the average

lifetime of a *hypothetical* cohort of people. Suppose that the age-specific death rates that occurred in Mexico in 1976 were to continue *unchanged* in all following years, until all the people born in Mexico in 1976 had died. Then the mean lifetime of this cohort would be (approximately) the *expectation of life at birth* for Mexico for 1976. It is not the average lifetime of the real cohort born in 1976, because age-specific death rates do change over time. But this expectation can be calculated from the 1976 age-specific death rates.* This use of a hypothetical cohort allows length of life, a fundamentally *longitudinal* concept, to be used to measure the *cross-sectional* idea of mortality in a *single* year, without allowing age structure to confuse the picture.

In Mexico in 1976 the expectation of life at birth was about 63 years for men and about 67 for women. The corresponding figures for England and Wales were: 69.7 years for men and 75.8 for women. These reflect the earlier findings from the age-specific death rates: in both countries male mortality is higher than female, but in Mexico mortality is higher than in England and Wales.

The concept of expectation of life at birth can be extended to expectation of life at other ages. For instance, the 1976 England and Wales figure for male expectation of life at birth is the mean length of life of the birth cohort of males born in 1976 if age-specific death rates do not change. But consider the cohort of males born in, say, 1931, who are aged 45 in 1976. What impact would the 1976 age-specific death rates have on them, assuming again that these rates do not change? The rates can be used to calculate the expectation of life at age 45 for England and Wales in 1976, which is the mean number of extra years which men aged 45 in 1976 would live if age-specific death rates did not change. In fact, this figure turned out to be 27.8 years.

□ Given that this cohort is aged 45, that seems to imply that their average age at death is 45 + 27.8 or 72.8 years. But the male expectation of life at birth in the same year in the same country was only 69.7 years. Can you explain this discrepancy? (Think about people who die before they are 45.)

■ The expectation of life at birth is a mean lifetime of the *whole* of a cohort, including those who die before the age of 45. The expectation of life at age 45 is the mean number of extra years lived by those who have actually reached 45 — the calculation *excludes* those who died before 45. So the average age of this 'part-cohort' will be greater than the mean lifetime of the whole cohort.

---

* Actually, the calculations are made on the basis that the chance of dying at any particular age remains constant. If the calculations were done on the basis of constant age-specific death rates, the result would differ, though only slightly.

In this discussion of mortality, we started by merely counting all deaths, and went on to look at age structure — which involved knowing the age at which people died. What other aspects of death are important to demographers and epidemiologists?

In birth registration in Britain, the only information recorded about the baby itself it its name, sex, date and place of birth. (The other information refers to the baby's parents.) But in death registration, more information is gathered. The age and occupation of the dead person, and where they lived are recorded. But a key piece of information recorded, which keeps many medical statisticians and epidemiologists in business, is the *cause of death*. For most deaths, this information comes from a death certificate completed by a doctor who attended the deceased during his or her last illness. Figure 5.5 shows the certificate used in England and Wales.

The doctor fills in the 'cause of death' box in the middle of the form, which is eventually sent to the Office of Population Censuses and Surveys (OPCS) in London. There, trained coders convert the information in the box into a number referring to one of the causes on a list called the International Classification of Diseases, Injuries and Causes of Death. These are generally known as ICD numbers. (As an example of the kind of cause given on the ICD list, 'cancer of the trachea, bronchus and lung' is ICD number 162 on the ninth revision of the International Classification, the version in use at the time of writing. The trachea is the 'windpipe' that carries air past the larynx (voice box) into the chest cavity, and the bronchi are the smaller pipes carrying air from the trachea into the lungs.)

Knowing what people died of is clearly going to be of more use to most health researchers than merely knowing how many people died of all causes put together. But as usual, the extra information comes at a cost of potential inaccuracy. If you were guillotined by the State, the cause of your death would be easy to determine and classify. (In fact, the cause of death could come under two headings: E978 legal execution and 806 fracture of vertebral column with spinal cord lesion.) But think about an old man, who has problems with many of his bodily systems. When he dies, his doctor must judge which of the diseases he suffered from caused his death, and which were merely subsidiary. This judgement is not straightforward. Several studies, both in the UK and the USA, have shown that the cause given on the death certificate is often different from that derived from the person's hospital case notes or the findings of a post-mortem. There may be discrepancies in as many as 30–50 per cent of cases. Afterwards, the OPCS coder has to convert what might be a considerable amount of information on the death certificate into a single ICD number. Studies conducted by the World Health Organization indicate that, although coders within a single country are pretty consistent in the way they produce these codes,

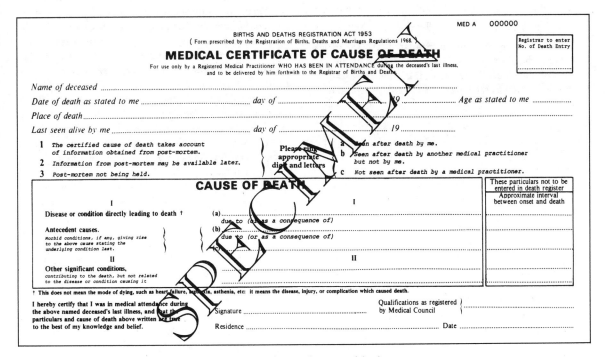

Figure 5.5 The central portion of the death certificate, which gives the cause of death.

there can be severe inconsistencies between coders from different countries. So the recording and coding of the cause of death is by no means an entirely objective process.

Despite the many problems associated with recording the cause of death, it is possible to calculate and use meaningful death rates from a particular cause, provided these problems are borne in mind when interpreting the resulting data. In 1980, 35 168 people in England and Wales were recorded as dying of lung cancer (including tracheal and bronchial cancers, ICD 162). So the crude death rate *from this cause* per thousand in 1980 was

$$\frac{\text{number of deaths from lung cancer}}{\text{total population}} \times 1\,000 = \frac{35\,168}{49\,244\,300} \times 1\,000.$$

$$= 0.714$$

Rather than dealing with small numbers like this, it is customary to calculate death rates from particular causes per hundred thousand (or per million) instead of per thousand. The crude death rate from lung cancer per hundred thousand for England and Wales 1980 was

$$\frac{35\,168}{49\,244\,300} \times 100\,000 = 71.4.$$

With many causes of death, it is valuable to look at the two sexes separately. For men, the crude death rate from lung cancer in England and Wales in 1980 was 111.7 (per hundred thousand). The corresponding rate per hundred thousand for women was 33.1, a much lower figure.

☐ In 1980, there were an estimated 277 000 males living in the county of Cleveland in the industrial north-east of England. There were 371 male lung cancer deaths. What was the lung cancer death rate for males?

■ It was

$$\frac{371}{277\,000} \times 100\,000,$$

or 133.9 per hundred thousand.

☐ The corresponding lung cancer death rate for males living in East Sussex (on the south coast) was 140.9 per hundred thousand. Does this mean lung cancer was a more severe problem in East Sussex than in Cleveland? (Think about what you know of the age of the people that live in the industrial north-east and on the south coast.)

■ On one hand, lung cancer does appear to be more of a problem in East Sussex. But the victims of lung cancer tend to be middle-aged or older. You may know that the population of areas like East Sussex contains more than its share of older people, many of whom have moved to the coast on retirement. People in

counties such as Cleveland tend to be younger. So perhaps the high lung cancer death rate in East Sussex merely reflects the fact that its population is older, and does not indicate that lung cancer is more prevalent there.

So age may be important too. As with the example of Mexico and England and Wales, the age structure of the populations must be considered. This can be done in various ways; for example, we could calculate age-specific death rates for lung cancer for both counties. But suppose we want just *one* figure for each sex. Although variations on the idea of life expectancy can be used, they are more difficult to interpret when considering deaths from a particular cause rather than all deaths. An alternative is to use what is known as *age standardisation*. To do this one needs to choose a *standard population* for reference. When one is looking at death rates in parts of a country, the population of the whole country is often a useful standard population to choose.

The main method of age standardisation you will meet here involves calculating the *standardised mortality ratio* (SMR). To arrive at the SMR one would use age-specific death rates for the standard population. So to work out the SMR for male deaths from lung cancer in Cleveland, using England and Wales as the standard, the first step would be to calculate the age-specific death rates for lung cancer for men in England and Wales. These can be used with the *Cleveland* population age structure to work out how many men *would have* died of lung cancer in Cleveland if the impact of the disease on men of any given age was the *same* as it was nationally. The number of men who actually did die of lung cancer in Cleveland is expressed as a percentage of this.

The male SMR for lung cancer in Cleveland in 1980 was 140. This is considerably over 100, which means that, on the whole, many more men (40 per cent more) died of lung cancer in Cleveland than might have been expected from the figures for England and Wales, allowing for differences in age structure.

The SMR for lung cancer for males in East Sussex in 1980 was only 91. This is less than 100, so fewer men died of lung cancer in East Sussex than might have been expected from the national figures. For some reason, lung cancer seems to be a more important cause of death in Cleveland than in East Sussex — the opposite of the conclusion you might draw from the crude death rates.

It is perhaps not quite obvious why the process of finding the SMR corrects for differences in age structure. But it is important to remember that it *does*, and that the bigger the SMR, the more deaths there are in the area being studied compared with the number one would expect from deaths in the standard population.

Calculating the SMR is not the only possible way of doing age standardisation. It is an example of what is known as *indirect standardisation*. There is a technique called *direct standardisation* as well, which is rather less used in the context of death rates.

The two methods tend to lead to similar conclusions; but if there are large differences in age structure or age-specific death rates the methods can produce different conclusions. So, which conclusions should be used? There is not really an answer to this; both methods involve reducing a whole list of age-specific death rates to a single number, and if the two methods disagree, the conclusion can only be that this process of reduction is not always appropriate.

All the previous examples have involved comparisons of mortality in different places at the same time, but the same techniques can be used to compare mortality in the same place at different times. In this instance, the standard population used for standardisation is generally the population at some time in the middle of the period being studied. Thus, the changing impact of a particular cause of death can be studied.

Figure 5.6 is taken from a Government document on the prevention of disease. It shows the SMR for tuberculosis in England and Wales over a century, taking the population in 1950–52 as the standard reference population. It purports to show that the introduction of certain preventive measures, and new drug treatment, earlier this century caused tuberculosis death rates to fall.

☐ Does the graph show this? (Look carefully at the scale on the vertical axis.)

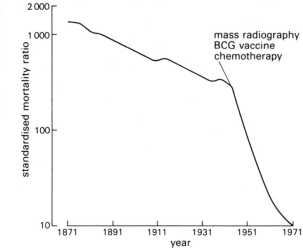

Figure 5.6 Age standardisation. The mortality from tuberculosis in England and Wales, 1871–1971. (redrawn from DHSS (1976) Figure 2.4)

■ Perhaps things are less clear than they look at first glance! The numbers on the vertical scale are not equally spaced. For example, the gap between 10 and 100 — an interval of 90 — is the same length as the interval of 900 between 100 and 1 000.

If the graph is drawn with a *linear* (evenly-spaced) *scale*, it looks like Figure 5.7. The impact of the new measures seems less marked in this figure. This is not to suggest that

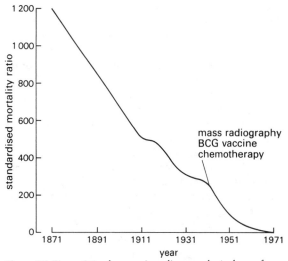

Figure 5.7 Figure 5.6 redrawn using a linear scale. (redrawn from Radical Statistics Health Group, 1976, Figure B)

the first graph is wrong — it has what is known as a *logarithmic* or *log scale* on the vertical axis, and there are often good reasons for using such a scale.* But you should look out for non-linear scales like this.

There can be difficulties in using SMRs, but the fact that they can correct for differences in population age structures and allow the comparison of 'like with like' makes them very useful — and widely used. (Similar techniques can be used to standardise for other differences in structure, for instance, differences in social class or occupation.) But again, the gain in usefulness has cost something in terms of the time and cost of collecting those data, and in potential accuracy. As well as knowing the number of deaths and the size of the population, one must know or estimate the age structure of the population being studied and the standard

---

* On the log scale, distance is proportional to the logarithm of the variable being measured, rather than just to the variable itself. If a variable is changing exponentially over time, so that it doubles (or halves) in equal periods of time, then a graph of its change over time with a logarithmic scale will produce a straight line, whose slope depends on the doubling (or halving) rate. This straight line can be easier to deal with than the curved graph that would arise if a linear scale were used.

population, and one must know the age at death of the people who died in the standard population (for indirect standardisation). These things are not always easy to measure or estimate. In demography, as with most other things, you get what you work for.

Of course, in an industrialised country like the UK a lot of the work is done routinely by government bodies. The Office of Population Censuses and Surveys (OPCS) publishes a wide range of mortality data, largely derived from the registration of deaths. These data include analyses by cause of death, age and sex; by cause of death and area of residence; and, every ten years in connection with the census, by cause of death and the occupation of the deceased. Regular publication of such data allows for the study of changes over time.

But OPCS data are not to be treated uncritically. Some of the problems of assigning and recording a cause of death have already been mentioned. Other problems arise with data on occupation. The next-of-kin reports the deceased person's last occupation; but this might not be what the person had worked at for most of their life, and what may have contributed to the cause of death. Indeed, the next-of-kin may not know, or remember, exactly what the dead person did at work.

Routine mortality statistics are produced in most industrialised and many Third World countries, but their accuracy and completeness varies considerably from one country to the next. Apart from questions of accuracy, there can be differences in the definitions used; for example, in France babies weighing less than 1 000 grams at birth are excluded from the calculation of the perinatal mortality rate. The World Health Organization and the United Nations produce weighty volumes annually, containing digests of demographic and mortality data from as many countries as possible.

Measuring disease

Epidemiologists study health and disease in populations, and we have just been discussing ways of measuring mortality in populations. But, luckily for the human race, not every illness kills. The great majority of episodes of illness end in recovery rather than death. So how can disease be measured in populations? Does it make any difference what the disease is?

First of all, try to compare counting instances of disease with counting deaths. There are three important differences.

1 It is, relatively speaking, easy to define when a person is dead; it is much less easy to define when a person is ill. When is a cold a cold, and when is it just a sniffle? Does a person count as having lung cancer when he or she feels ill, but has not yet had the disease diagnosed?

2 Deaths are (almost) all registered officially, in developed countries at any rate. Some diseases have to be officially notified in Britain — mainly certain infectious diseases such as measles, though in practice very many of these illnesses are not reported. In addition, there are some voluntary schemes for registering other diseases — notably cancers, where registration is thought to be around 70–80 per cent complete. But most episodes of disease are recorded only in the doctor's notes and hospital records — if the person gets as far as consulting a doctor.

3 Death occurs at a certain point in time, so it makes sense to talk about the time of death. A person suffers from a disease over a *period* of time — days, weeks, years.

The final point means that there can be two completely different counts of how common a disease is. First, one could count how many people *began* to suffer from the disease in a given period of time. This is the *incidence* of the disease. Second, one could count how many people actually had the disease at a given time. This is known as the *prevalence* of the disease.

Here is an analogous situation. A birth occurs at a given time, but the child lives on afterwards. So if a researcher was interested in mothers and children in 1983, two measures could be taken. First, the number of births in the year 1983 could be counted. Second, the number of mothers with children under, say, five on 30 June 1983 can be counted. Both of these would give some kind of measure of how common young children were, but they would differ.

As with births and deaths, to compare how common a given disease is in different places or at different times, it is necessary to compare the number of cases of the disease with the size of the population involved or, to be more precise, with the population at risk of having the disease. And as usual, this is done by calculating rates.

The *incidence rate* of a disease over a *period* of time is

$$\frac{\text{number of new cases over the period}}{\text{population at risk}}.$$

The *prevalence rate* of a disease at a *point* in time is

$$\frac{\text{total number of cases of the disease at that time}}{\text{population at risk}}.$$

Both these rates are generally expressed as percentages, or as rates per thousand or per hundred thousand.

As an example, suppose that in a certain (imaginary) town the following data were recorded.

1 Number of new cases of diabetes in the year 1977 was 289.

2 Total number of sufferers from diabetes on 30 June 1977 was 3 492.

3 Population in 1977 was 176 000.

So the incidence rate per 100 000 for this disease in 1977 was

$$\frac{289}{176\,000} \times 100\,000 = 164.2.$$

The prevalence rate on 30 June 1977 was

$$\frac{3\,492}{176\,000} \times 100\,000 = 1\,984.1.$$

☐   In the imaginary town (population 176 000) there were 4 500 new cases of influenza in 1977, and the total number of sufferers from this disease on 30 June 1977 was 60. What were the corresponding incidence and prevalence rates per 100 000?

■   The incidence rate for 1977 was

$$\frac{4\,500}{176\,000} \times 100\,000 = 2\,556.8 \text{ per } 100\,000.$$

The prevalence rate on 30 June 1977 was

$$\frac{60}{176\,000} \times 100\,000 = 34.1 \text{ per } 100\,000.$$

☐   For diabetes, the prevalence rate is considerably greater than the incidence rate. For influenza it is the other way round. Can you explain this?

■   Diabetes is a *chronic disease*; that is people usually suffer from it for many years. So the number of new cases in any year is small compared with the number of existing cases, and the incidence rate is smaller than the prevalence rate. Influenza is an *acute disease* and lasts a much shorter time (normally just a few days), so many more people catch it in a year than actually suffer from it at a given time, and the rates are the other way round.

Perhaps the main difficulty in using incidence and prevalence rates to measure disease is actually finding the data necessary to calculate them. Such data come from a number of different types of sources.

In Britain, routine statistics on illness, so-called *morbidity statistics*, are based mainly on the use of National Health Service facilities. Since 1952, the Hospital In-patient Enquiry (HIPE) has been in operation. This records various characteristics of one in every ten hospital in-patients. Another system, the Hospital Activity Analysis (HAA) was established in the 1970s and records demographic data on the patient (age, sex, residence, marital status), clinical data (diagnoses, operations) and administrative data for each episode of in-patient care. A limitation of these systems is that their statistics relate to episodes of care rather than to individual patients. If a person returns to hospital several times with the same illness, this will have the same impact on the statistics as if several people were admitted once each. This can clearly distort calculations of incidence and prevalence.

Some general practitioners — a self-selected sample — contribute to a national survey of GP consultations and episodes of illness run by the Royal College of General Practitioners. Results from this are published regularly (though infrequently), and provide, in particular, data on incidence rates.

A disadvantage of all these methods is that they cannot measure illness and disability that do not involve the health services. There are, however, sources of data that do not have this disadvantage. In particular, information on morbidity is sometimes derived from surveys of the population. Such surveys may be concerned with all types of illness, or they may concentrate on a particular disease or type of disability. They involve taking a representative sample of individuals from a particular population, and the incidence or prevalence of the illness (or illnesses) concerned can be measured in, essentially, two different ways. Either the people in the sample can be asked about their health — *self-assessment* — or biomedical tests can be carried out on them to indicate whether or not they are ill — *screening*.

The General Household Survey (GHS) conducted by OPCS is the main British example of self-assessment. The resulting data are published (together with data on many other topics) in the annual GHS reports.

An example of screening is provided by a survey carried out in Bedford in the 1960s to investigate the prevalence of diabetes. A randomly chosen sample was taken of people of all ages, well or ill, living in the town. These people were given a standard test used to diagnose diabetes, which involved the measurement of the amount of sugar in the blood some time after they had eaten a measured amount of sugar. Straightforward, you might think. But in fact there is no general agreement on exactly where the line should be drawn between 'normal' blood sugar levels and the 'abnormally high' levels that indicate diabetes. Certainly, all diabetics do not have one blood sugar level and everyone else another. In the Bedford study, the number counted as having diabetes ranged between 7 per cent and 32 per cent of the sample, depending on where the line was drawn. Certainly it was not true that 32 per cent, or even 7 per cent, of the people in the sample *knew* they had diabetes.

Apart from such problems of defining and diagnosing who has a particular illness, surveys that use a sample of the population raise another question. How can one be sure that what is observed in the sample accurately reflects what is happening in the whole population from which the sample was drawn? Using one criterion, 7 per cent of the Bedford sample were diagnosed as diabetic, but does this mean that 7 per cent of the entire *population* of Bedford would be diagnosed as having diabetes under this criterion?

In other words, is the sample *representative* of the population? Whether or not it is depends on how large the sample is, and how it was chosen.

If you wanted to predict the outcome of a forthcoming general election, it would clearly be inadequate to ask the members of your local Conservative club who they were going to vote for. That sample would not be representative. Your sample should, ideally, include people from all parts of the country, of all ages and both sexes, of all degrees of prosperity, and so on. Choosing such a sample would probably involve selecting people *at random* from a list of electors — in Chapter 6 you will see why. Even if you did this, a sample of, say, twenty electors would not be enough; but you would not need to go to the other extreme and select a sample of several million. Political opinion polls produce reasonably accurate predictions of voting behaviour from samples of a few thousand, or even fewer.

This question of inferring what is going on in a population from measurements made on a sample has been widely studied by statisticians, and will come up later, in Chapter 6 and again in Chapter 10. For now, all you need to remember is that in general, provided the sample is chosen in a satisfactory way and is sufficiently large, it *is* possible to make reasonably accurate inferences of this type. In summary, surveys can provide very useful information about illness in a population, but as always, care must be taken in interpreting this information.

In this chapter, you have learned about ways of measuring some of the demographic characteristics of a population, as well as about the impact of different diseases and causes of death. In the next chapter, we shall introduce some of the methods used by epidemiologists and clinicians to establish the causes of disease, and evaluate methods of treatment and prevention.

Objectives of Chapter 5

When you have studied this chapter, you should be able to:

5.1 Broadly define the field of study of demography and epidemiology, and outline the basic methods of inquiry of demography.

5.2 Define the terms: crude birth rate, general fertility rate, crude death rate, incidence and prevalence rates, and calculate them from given data.

5.3 Describe the process of registering births and deaths, and the production of fertility, mortality, and morbidity statistics in the UK and outline the limitations of these statistics.

5.4 Exemplify the need to consider the age and sex structure of populations when investigating fertility and mortality.

5.5 Define, in general terms, the following: age-specific death rate, expectation of life, standardised mortality ratio; and interpret statements that use these concepts.

Questions for Chapter 5

1 (*Objective 5.1*) Which of the following would epidemiologists be particularly interested in?

(i) the number of deaths in Scotland in 1983

(ii) the number of deaths from burns in Scotland in 1983

(iii) the fact that Mr Lawson (Chapter 2) had diabetes

(iv) the data on smoking and lung cancer, which you met in question 4 of the last chapter (p.34).

2 (*Objective 5.2*) In Scotland in 1980, there were 68 892 live births and 63 299 deaths in an estimated population of 5 153 300. The number of women aged 15–44 was estimated as 1 080 600. Calculate: (a) the crude birth rate; (b) the crude death rate; and (c) the general fertility rate for Scotland in 1980.

3 (*Objectives 5.1 and 5.3*) Mrs Wells was elderly and ill. Her doctors diagnosed stomach cancer, and when she died, they considered that the cancer had been the main cause of her death. Describe how this information eventually gets into the published mortality statistics.

4 (*Objectives 5.4 and 5.5*) The data on lung cancer in occupational groups, which you met in question 4 for Chapter 4, gave the SMR for lung cancer for each occupational group. The standard population was that for the whole of England and Wales.

(a) Why use the SMR rather than the crude lung cancer death rate for each group?

(b) In these data, construction workers had a SMR for lung cancer of 144, whereas sales workers had an SMR of 85. What do these figures mean?

5 (*Objective 5.5*) On p.42 you learned that the expectation of life of 45-year-old males in England and Wales in 1976 was 27.8 years. A man aged 45 in 1976 was born in 1931, when the expectation of life at birth was 58.7 years. Give *two* reasons why this figure is less than 45 + 27.8.

6 (*Objective 5.2*) In a certain town, the population was 56 300 in 1982. There were 119 sufferers from multiple sclerosis on 30 June that year. During the year, 5 new cases of the disease were diagnosed. What are (a) the incidence and (b) the prevalence rates for multiple sclerosis in that town for 1982?

6

Investigating causes and evaluating treatments

This chapter contains references to the Course Reader, so you should have it to hand as you work. You will be asked to read articles by Smithells *et al.* (1980) and Laurence *et al.* (1981), reprinted in Part 3, Section 3.6. You could look at the rest of the material in this section on ethical dilemmas in evaluation if you have time, but we shall come back to the question of ethics later in the course.

Much of the teaching in this chapter is illustrated by reference to neural-tube defects including spina bifida. More details of the biology of such defects are given in Book IV, *The Biology of Health and Disease*, but you should remember that, as with diabetes in Chapter 2, you are not expected to remember specific features of this disorder.

If you are familiar with statistical hypothesis testing and confidence intervals, you will find that you already know much of the material on pp.52–4; even so, we advise you to look quickly through that section and to check your grasp of the material by working through the objectives and questions at the end of the chapter.

Epidemiology uses many methods to investigate why people suffer from disease. At the beginning of Chapter 5 you met Snow's work on cholera; he used the simple, but often powerful, technique of plotting the location of cases of a disease on a map. Then there were several examples of data from officially published statistics — epidemiologists often use these in their work. Now we shall look at some of the types of epidemiological study that investigate causes of disease.

You have probably heard of spina bifida. It is a disorder that arises during fetal development in which the backbone, and the spinal cord it contains, do not develop properly. Babies born with this condition *may* be relatively unaffected, but many of them are severely handicapped. In biological terms, spina bifida can occur when something goes wrong in part of the developing fetus called the neural tube: for this reason, spina bifida and other related disorders are collectively known as *neural-tube defects*.*

It has been estimated that in England and Wales in 1980, a neural-tube defect was present in just under two in every thousand births.

Many different explanations of neural-tube defects have been put forward. These defects are much more common in some geographical areas than others — over twice as common in Northern Ireland than in London, for example. In some areas (though not all) neural-tube defects are considerably less common among wealthier families than in those that are less well off. These observations could provide the basis for an explanation of neural-tube defects.

* More details of the biology of neural-tube defects are given in *The Biology of Health and Disease*. (U205, Book IV)

□ Can you think of any characteristic of people, or of what they do, that varies from place to place, and from one social class to another within the same area, that might possibly lead to neural-tube defects?

■ There are numerous possibilities. One is smoking — people smoke more in some parts of the country than in others, and manual workers and their families smoke more than white-collar workers. Something in the smoke could quite possibly affect a developing fetus. (But in fact there is no evidence that this is so: the babies of mothers who smoke do not seem to be particularly prone to neural-tube defects, although other adverse effects *have* been attributed to smoking during pregnancy.)

Another possible cause, which several investigators have looked at, is diet. Again, this varies from place to place and across social classes, and it is plausible that what a mother eats, or does not eat during pregnancy, could affect her baby.

How might one investigate the theory that neural-tube defects have something to do with the mother's diet during pregnancy? One way to start would be to look at the diets of mothers who have given birth to babies with neural-tube defects. Suppose this research were undertaken and it was found that 60 per cent of the mothers studied had eaten no spring greens.

□ Can you conclude from this that failure to eat spring greens during pregnancy increases the risk of this condition?

■ No. There are many reasons why not, but the most important of these is the lack of other babies for *comparison*. You would also need to know what the mothers of perfectly healthy babies had been eating during pregnancy. It may be that 60 per cent of them also never ate spring greens. If so, the answer seems unlikely to lie in this particular aspect of diet. On the other hand, if over 90 per cent of the mothers of healthy babies say they did eat spring greens, then you may be onto something important.

Such comparative studies are technically known as *case-control studies*. In a case-control study, a group of *cases* — or sufferers from the disease in question — is identified. Another group of *controls*, or people who do not have the disease, is then found. The idea is to find a group of controls who are similar to the cases, apart from the fact that they do not have the disease being studied. Most case-control studies are *retrospective*. A study is said to be retrospective if it looks back into the personal history of the people being studied and investigates things that happened before they were under study.

Much research on the causes of neural-tube defects has been carried out by K. M. Laurence (a paediatrician and geneticist) and his colleagues, based in Cardiff. One of their studies (Laurence *et al.*, 1980) used just such a case-control method; the cases were babies born with a neural-tube defect in South Wales, and the controls were babies who had been born to the same mothers but had not suffered from neural-tube defects. The mothers were asked about their diet during the 'case' and the 'control' pregnancies; these diets were classified as being 'good', 'fair' or 'poor'. ('Good' diets were varied, balanced, and considered to provide an ample supply of important nutrients.) It turned out that the mothers' diets during 'case' pregnancies were on average, rather worse than their diets during 'control' pregnancies.

□ Does this *show* that a poor diet (as defined in this study) increases a mother's chance of having a child affected by a neural-tube defect? (Think about how *you* might react if you had one child that was affected and one that was not, and a doctor who was studying neural-tube defects asked you about your diet in the two pregnancies.)

■ The result certainly lends support to the hypothesis of a dietary cause, but it does not prove it. One important difficulty is that the mother may *think* about her diets in the two pregnancies differently, even if they were identical, just because the pregnancies had different outcomes. For example, if the mother suspected that diet affects the chance of having a baby with a neural-tube defect, she might be more likely to report that her diet was worse during the pregnancy that produced the affected child.

This kind of difficulty is very often present with data collected retrospectively. If it is already known who got the disease and who did not, there is always a chance that this knowledge can bias the investigations. Of course, it is not possible to tell in the Laurence study whether this bias *was* present, but it is possible that it was, and this has to be borne in mind when the results are interpreted.

A later study by the Cardiff group (James *et al.*, 1980) demonstrates another difficulty in interpreting retrospective case-control studies, though this time the difficulty stems from the case-control part, not from the retrospective nature of the study (in fact, strictly speaking, the study was not retrospective at all, as you will see). This time the cases were mothers who had had babies with neural-tube defects in South Wales, and the controls were the sisters of these mothers, who had not had affected babies. The women were asked about their present diet rather than about their diet during pregnancy. (This reduces, though it does not remove, the problem of bias in what the mothers recall about their past diet; but it introduces a new problem, that a mother's diet may have changed since the pregnancy.) Table 6.1 summarises some of the data from this study.

Table 6.1 Quality of mother's diet in a case-control study of neural-tube defects in South Wales

Group of women	Quality of diet			Row total
	good	fair	poor	
cases	34	110	100	244
controls (sisters)	43	48	32	123

(data from James *et al.*, 1980, p.305)

☐ Summarise in words what this table shows.

■ The cases tend to have worse diets than the controls.

If this is not obvious, it is worth working out the row percentages (Table 6.2).

Table 6.2 Quality of mother's diet in a case-control study of neural-tube defects in South Wales (row percentages)

Group of women	Quality of diet			Total (= 100%)
	good	fair	poor	
Cases	13.9	45.1	41.0	244
controls (sisters)	35.0	39.0	26.0	123

This makes it easier to see that, for example, far more of the controls (35 per cent) had a good diet than did the cases (13.9 per cent).

☐ Does *this* prove that a poor diet during pregnancy tends to cause neural-tube defects? (Think about other ways in which the cases might differ from the controls.)

■ Again the data tend to support this, but perhaps the cases and controls differed in some way *other* than diet, and it may be this other difference that causes neural-tube defects in the cases. So there is room for doubt.

Such doubt arises from the nature of case-control studies, which depend for their validity on the cases and controls being comparable in all respects, apart from the presence of the disease (in the cases). However, as you can imagine, the process of checking for *all* possible differences between cases and controls is impossible. In practice this process of checking is restricted to those factors that the investigators believe *may* affect the disease being studied. Although such a restriction is clearly essential on practical grounds, it does mean that a case-control study can never *prove* or *disprove* a causal hypothesis, but can only demonstrate an *association*.

Case-control studies all suffer from the fact that any difference observed between the cases and the controls *may* be due to the way the controls were chosen rather than having anything to do with the disease in question.

There is a different kind of study that avoids some of the problems of case-control studies. For example, a researcher might select a group of mothers at the start of their pregnancy (or even before), record their eating habits during pregnancy, and eventually record whether their babies had neural-tube defects. This avoids problems of matching cases and controls, *and* the fact that the outcome of the pregnancy may influence the way in which diet is reported. This is a *prospective cohort study*. In such a study, a group of people is chosen *before* any have the disease being studied. They are then followed up into the future, and their exposure to potential causes of the disease is recorded. Eventually, some of them will contract the disease, and the chance of contracting it can be compared for different levels of exposure to the possible causes. It is called a *prospective* study because instead of looking back at personal history that has already occurred, the study follows people forward through time. It is a *cohort* study because those being studied form a *cohort*; that is, they share a common experience — in this instance being pregnant at about the same time and in the same area. (Remember the cohorts you met in the last chapter, for example, all those *born* in a particular place (e.g. Mexico) in a particular year.)

It is possible to carry out other types of study, such as a retrospective cohort study.

☐ How would you go about setting up a retrospective cohort study?

■ A *cohort* of people would be chosen on the basis of their *previous* exposure to, or experience of, the factor under study, regardless of whether or not they had the disease in question. One would then record whether they did have the disease, and go *back* into their personal histories to look for potential causes. Retrospective cohort studies have been used, for example, to investigate the possible risks to health of working in plants dealing with the production and reprocessing of nuclear fuel. Cohorts of people who worked in such plants in the past have been compared with people who worked elsewhere, to measure the extent to which the ex-nuclear workers were more likely to have developed diseases such as cancer.

The main disadvantages of a prospective study compared with a retrospective one are that it usually takes longer to carry out and may cost much more. In the study of diet during pregnancy, this may not be too important, as pregnancy lasts only nine months. But prospective studies of, for example, potential causes of cancer may run for decades, because the disease may not become apparent until long after the exposure to the factor suspected of making the disease more likely. A retrospective study can be done much more rapidly and cheaply.

The main problem in using a cohort study rather than a case-control study lies in the number of people one has to study. Cohort studies can require far more people, if the disease being studied is relatively uncommon.

For example, neural-tube defects affect roughly one baby in 500 in England and Wales; to end up with an adequate number of affected infants to study, you would need to have a huge number of pregnant mothers in the cohort. To find 50 affected babies, you would need about 25 000 women. In a case-control study, you would need to study only the 50 affected babies and a relatively small number of controls to compare them with — perhaps another 50, though a study of this nature might well use more controls than this. Two per case, or 100 in all, might be used.

Because of these problems, prospective cohort studies tend to be much more expensive in time and money than retrospective case-control or cohort studies — so the retrospective studies are much more common. One way of reducing the number of people studied and the cost of cohort studies is to concentrate on a group of people known to be at high risk. Women who have already had a pregnancy affected by a neural-tube defect are more likely to have another. The Cardiff workers followed up their retrospective studies with prospective cohort studies that investigated the question: 'Does poor diet cause mothers who have already had a neural-tube defect pregnancy to be more likely to have another?' Some of the results from the prospective part of the second study are given in Table 6.3.

All these mothers had previously had affected babies, so they were all 'cases' in Tables 6.1 and 6.2. Overall, their diet was better than that of the cases in Tables 6.1 and 6.2. (They had received counselling to improve their diet.)

☐ What does Table 6.3 show?
■ All the recurrences of neural-tube defects were to mothers whose diet had been poor in early pregnancy. This gives support to the view that a poor diet during pregnancy is associated with neural-tube defects.

However, there is another important point to take into account. One of the main reasons for studying diet and neural-tube defects is to find a way of preventing such defects in the future. If you look at the 176 women in Table

6.3 in isolation, there is clearly an association between poor diet and the recurrence of neural-tube defects. But what would have happened if more women had been included in the study? Would the results have been the same? The 176 women in the study can be regarded as a sample from the population of women in South Wales who may be at risk of having a recurrence of neural-tube defects, now, in the past, or in the future. What do the results from the sample tell us about the population?

Dealing with chance

In terms of this population, there are two possible explanations of what the Cardiff team observed in their sample. First, perhaps there really is an association between poor diet and the recurrence of neural-tube defects that is reflected in the sample and requires further investigation. Second, perhaps there is *no* such association in the population, and the sample results look as they do by chance. It might just be a coincidence that all the recurrences occurred in the group of women whose diet was poor. (Think about shuffling a pack of playing cards and dealing out a sample of four of them. Suppose all four cards in the sample are kings. This might be because the pack (the population) is not of the usual kind and includes more than its share of kings, or it might just be a coincidence. Even with perfectly ordinary packs of cards, four kings in a row are dealt sometimes.) Before concluding that the sample results do indicate an association in the population, it is necessary to investigate whether the sample results were just a coincidence.

☐ Suppose that there were no association between poor diet and the recurrence of neural-tube defects in the population as a whole. Do you think it would be *likely* that results like those in Table 6.3 could be obtained from a sample of 176 women from the population?
■ You probably thought that results as extreme as those in the table would be very unlikely, if the supposition of no association in the population were true.

Table 6.3 Mother's diet and the outcome of pregnancy in a prospective study of neural-tube defects in South Wales

Outcome of pregnancy	Diet during first three months of pregnancy			Row total
	good	fair	poor	
normal	68	76	27	171
neural-tube defect	0	0	5	5

(data from James *et al.*, 1980, p.305)

□ What would you conclude about the supposition therefore?

■ It is unlikely to be true. That is, it seems that poor diet and the recurrence of neural-tube defects *are* associated in the population.

What you have done here is analogous to the following argument:

Supposition All birds can fly.

Observation Here is an ostrich. It is a bird. It cannot fly.

Reasoning The observation is inconsistent with the supposition. So the supposition must be wrong.

Conclusion It is not true that all birds can fly. Some birds cannot fly.

The difference between this and the argument about neural-tube defects is that in the latter, things are not so clear-cut. That argument goes:

Supposition Diet and the recurrence of neural-tube defects are *not* associated in the population.

Observation The data in Table 6.3 were collected.

Reasoning The observation is not completely inconsistent with the supposition. But it is very unlikely that an observation as extreme as this would have been made, if the supposition were true. So doubt is cast on the supposition.

Conclusion The supposition is probably wrong. There probably is an association between diet and the recurrence of neural-tube defects in the population.

This method of reaching conclusions about a population on the basis of data from a sample follows the general lines of a statistical *significance test*. The key step in the argument is the remark that, if the supposition of no association were true, then results as extreme as those obtained would be unlikely; and it is this step that is formalised in significance testing.

To carry out this formalisation, it is necessary to attach a number to statements such as, 'It is very unlikely that an observation as extreme as this would have been made, if the supposition of no association is true.' Exactly how unlikely is it? The scale used is called *probability*. On this scale, an event that cannot occur at all — as unlikely as can be — is given a probability of 0. An event that is certain to occur is given a probability of 1. Anything between — which might or might not occur — has a probability between 0 and 1. The more likely it is to occur, the higher the probability. If you toss a coin, it is just as likely that a head will come up as a tail. That is, a head is as likely as not, so that the event 'head comes up' has a probability halfway along the scale from 0 to 1; its probability is 1/2 or 0.5. Thinking of this in another way, there is one chance in two (1/2) that a head will come up. Similarly, there is one chance in six of throwing a two on a dice — the probability is 1/6.

We do not expect you to be able to *perform* a significance test yourself. Different significance tests are used in different situations, but they follow the same general method:

1 Begin with a *supposition* that the effect or association you are looking for is *not there* in the population. That is, suppose that any association in the sample is there purely by chance. (This supposition is usually called the null hypothesis — 'null' because it assumes no association.)

2 Work out (or, more often, look up in a special table) the probability of getting results at least as extreme as those actually *observed*, if the supposition of no association is true.

3 If this probability is small enough, then the results obtained are unlikely under the supposition of no association. This casts doubt on the supposition — so it is rejected, and the conclusion is that the effect or association you are looking for *does* exist in the population.

You will see later what happens if the probability calculated in step 2 is *not* small enough to reject the null hypothesis. But, first of all, let us return to the Cardiff study. Referring to the data in Table 6.3, the researchers reported that 'This distribution [of neural-tube defect recurrences] was unlikely to have occurred by chance ($P < 0.01$).' (Laurence *et al.*, 1983, p.91) That is, they had carried out an appropriate significance test, and had calculated that *if* diet and the recurrence of neural-tube defects were not associated in the population, then the probability (P) of getting a result as extreme as theirs was less than ($<$) one in a hundred ($0.01 = 1/100$). Therefore, they rejected the null hypothesis of no association and concluded that poor diet and the recurrence of neural-tube defects *were* associated in the population. (You should bear in mind that this argument is necessarily based on probabilities; so there is a small but unavoidable chance that the conclusion is wrong.)

Laurence and his colleagues took the view that a probability of less than 0.01 was sufficiently small to reject the explanation of their data that suggested the results were solely due to chance. Most people would agree with them — but what if their results had been less clear-cut and the if probability had been larger? There is a strong convention that a probability of less than 0.05 is small enough to reject the null hypothesis, whereas anything larger than 0.05 is not small enough. This corresponds to one chance in 20, because $1/20 = 0.05$. It is also referred to as a 5 per cent significance level — 5 per cent because $0.05 = 5/100$, and a result that gives a probability of 0.05 or less is said to be (statistically) significant at the 5 per cent level. (This use of the word 'significant' has nothing to do with medical or biological significance.) However, using a 5 per cent significance level is only a convention, and is not always sensible. For example, in a situation where more caution is called for, a smaller significance level — perhaps 1 per cent — may well be more appropriate.

What happens if the results are not (statistically) significant; that is, the calculated probability is *not* less than 0.05 (or whatever significance level is being used)?

☐ Suppose the Cardiff researchers had obtained different data, and had calculated a probability of, say, 0.2 in their significance test. What should they have concluded?

■ On this result they could not have ruled out the null hypothesis, so it would have been quite possible that diet and the recurrence of neural-tube defects were not associated. (However, it would still be possible that there *was* such an association in the population.)

Particularly when small samples are involved, it can be unwarranted to conclude that the null hypothesis is true just because it is not rejected. (It is usually possible to perform calculations of what is known as the *power* of a significance test, which throw light on this question. Most statisticians recommend that this is done before conclusions are drawn when a null hypothesis is not rejected; but in practice this advice is not often followed.) So, usually, 'results not significant' means 'we have not ruled out the explanation that the observed results are purely due to chance'; it does not mean this chance explanation is the *only* plausible one.

In this discussion we have concentrated on significance testing because it is the method of drawing conclusions from a sample most commonly used in biomedical and social research. But it is certainly not the only technique available. Rather than asking whether diet has any effect on the chance of recurrence of neural tube defects, it may well be more useful to ask how large an effect it has. This cannot be answered with a significance test. A wide range of techniques of *estimation* is available to deal with questions like this. For example, in the Cardiff study, 5 out of 32 mothers on a poor diet had a recurrence of a neural-tube defect. In other words, the rate of recurrence for mothers in the sample was 15.6 per cent ($5/27 \times 100 = 18.5$). But this does not mean that the rate of recurrence in the *population* of all mothers on a poor diet will be 15.6 per cent. In fact, it can be calculated that any value between 7 per cent and 32 per cent would be a plausible rate of recurrence in the population, on the basis of this sample. (Because the sample is fairly small, the range is wide.) This range of values is known as a *confidence interval* for the rate — actually a 95 per cent confidence interval because there is a probability of 0.95 that a confidence interval calculated this way does include the true rate for the population. Confidence intervals are used less than they could be in analysing biomedical and epidemiological data, and most statisticians would probably agree that they should be used more. However, they do not play an important role in our discussion of health and disease.

Intervention trials

Let us return again to the data from the Cardiff study, given in Table 6.3. You have seen that one can be reasonably certain that their results were not simply due to chance; the association is very likely to exist in the population from which these women were drawn.

☐ Can one *now* conclude that a poor diet during pregnancy causes an increase in the chance of having a baby with a neural-tube defect?

■ No, because as we mentioned before, the association may not be causal. Some other factor may be causing some mothers to eat poorly and, independently, causing the recurrence of neural-tube defects.

☐ Suppose the association between diet and neural-tube defects *were* due to a third factor like this. Could the recurrence of neural-tube defects be prevented or reduced by improving diet?

■ Not necessarily, because the third factor would not necessarily be changed by this improvement in diet.

So, it is important to consider whether an association is causal or not before proposing an intervention — a method of preventing, curing or alleviating the disease in question. In the study of maternal diet, a non-causal association would mean that the groups of women who had different diets differed also in some other way — in terms of the unknown third factor. If it could be arranged that the groups of women differed *only* in their diet, then a third-factor explanation would be ruled out, and one could be more confident in concluding that poor diet caused the recurrence of neural-tube defects. But it is extremely unlikely that two groups of women who happened to have different standards of diet would *not* differ in any other way. In any study that relies solely on *observing* mothers' diets (as did the case-control and cohort studies you met earlier in the chapter) such third-factor explanations cannot be ruled out.

If you were a cruel dictator, however, you could get out of this problem. You could take a group of pregnant women that was as homogeneous as possible. You could split it into two groups and feed one group on a good diet and one on a poor diet, and see what happened. This time, if the group with a poor diet produced more neural-tube defects, you would be fairly safe in concluding that poor diet had caused the defects. But such an action would probably not be ethically acceptable in our society (though you will recall from Chapter 3 that studies of this general nature *were* done by Goldberger in investigating dietary causes of pellagra). What are the alternatives? It *might* be considered ethically acceptable to carry out an experiment like this on animals; but a deeper biological understanding of what is involved would be needed in order to decide whether the results could be applied to humans. But ethical problems do not rule out *all* experiments with humans.

Studies such as those in South Wales, and some work with animals, led some researchers to consider it possible that it was not poor diet *in general* that increased the chance of a neural-tube defect, but that the defect was caused by a deficiency of a particular vitamin, folic acid. They thought that women who did not take in sufficient folic acid in their food during early pregnancy might be more likely to have an affected baby.

☐ If this hypothesis were true, what implications would it have for preventing neural-tube defects?

■ If pregnant women were given extra folic acid, either by improving their diet or by giving them folic acid pills, then there would be fewer neural-tube defects.

The problem is to decide whether such an intervention really does work. Again, most of the studies conducted so far have been concerned with the effect of this sort of intervention on the *recurrence* of neural-tube defects in mothers who have already had one affected child.

☐ Suppose you gave extra folic acid to such a mother, and her next baby was not affected. What does this tell you?

■ Not much. The chances are that the baby would not have been affected anyway.

☐ What if you gave folic acid to a thousand such mothers, and only ten had an affected child?

■ This would provide *some* evidence, but you still do not know how many of them would have had babies with neural-tube defects *without* the folic acid.

What is needed is a *control* group — a group of mothers who do not receive the extra folic acid, but are otherwise as similar as possible to the first group. Then, if fewer of the mothers in the group receiving extra folic acid had affected babies, and if the difference was large enough to be statistically significant, one could conclude that the intervention did have a useful result. This is an example of an *intervention trial*. It is an *experiment* — because the researcher intervenes and changes what would otherwise happen, rather than merely observing.

You might wonder why folic acid is not given to all pregnant women anyway. Unless there is acceptable evidence that the intervention actually works, this is inadvisable. As regards the woman's health, even though folic acid is a vitamin, it is conceivable that large doses of it may be harmful to health in some way. From the point of view of society, it would be wasteful to spend money on folic acid supplementation if it is ineffective. We shall return to these points later.

In the intervention trial we have just outlined, one group of women would receive folic acid and the others nothing, so the comparison is between folic acid treatment and no treatment. In other trials, a different comparison may be made. Suppose, for example, a new drug to treat high blood pressure were developed. Reasonably effective drugs for this condition already exist.

☐ Would it make sense to run an intervention trial in which some patients with high blood pressure got the new drug and the others got no treatment at all?

■ No, for two reasons. First, the patients who received no treatment would be worse off than if they were not in the trial — when they would receive an already existing treatment rather than nothing at all. This would not be considered ethically acceptable. Second, a researcher is much more likely to be interested in comparing the new drug with existing treatments, rather than with no treatment. The question asked will probably be, 'Is this drug any better than what is currently used?' rather than, 'Is this drug better than nothing?'

Most intervention trials, therefore, proceed by giving the treatment or intervention being studied to one group of people — the *experimental group* — and giving either an established treatment, or nothing at all, to another group — the *control group*. (This type of trial is said to be group-comparative because it compares two separate groups of individuals. There are other kinds of trial which are organised differently.) In a trial of this kind, if the results *are* to be used to investigate causal explanations rather than merely associations, the two groups must be as similar and homogeneous as possible in every way, other than the fact that they receive different treatments. This requirement imposes several limitations on the way an intervention trial is designed and run. Three things need to be specified precisely: the type of person to be studied, the treatment, and how the outcome will be measured.

First, it is important to specify exactly what type of person will be eligible for inclusion in the trial. In a trial of folic acid to prevent the recurrence of neural-tube defects, for example, only mothers who had previously had an affected baby would be included. Also the study might be limited further, say, to mothers in a particular age group. There is a balance to be struck between the homogeneity achieved by such *selection criteria* and the fact that such limitations also limit the applicability of the results. If all the mothers in the trial were aged between 20 and 25, then the conclusions of the trial could, strictly speaking, be applied only to mothers in this rather narrow age range. Some people will be included or excluded on practical grounds; there would be no point in including a mother who refused to take any pills, for example. The criteria used for inclusion or exclusion should be made clear in reports on the trial, so that readers can decide for themselves exactly where the results can be used.

Second, it is important to specify exactly what treatment will be given to the people in the two groups. It would be no good reading a report that said merely, 'One group had extra folic acid, and the other did not.' How much folic acid? When was it taken?

Another important point about treatments. Suppose the mothers in one group take a folic acid pill each day, and the others do not.

☐ Apart from the folic acid content of the pills, how do the groups differ?

■ The control group of mothers have not taken a pill.

This is not as silly as it sounds. Often, taking a pill without any active ingredients at all can have an effect on a person. Some illnesses can even be cured by such apparently inert pills, which are called *placebos*. This *placebo effect* is by no means confined to particularly credulous or suggestible people. So it is common practice, in trials where the experimental group receives a drug in pill or injection form and the control group gets no active treatment, to give the control group an inert placebo pill or injection. (Similar ideas have even been used in some trials of surgical procedures — the controls had a brief general anaesthetic and even a shallow incision in their bodies — though some people would question whether this is ethically acceptable.) If a trial is designed so that the patients are unaware which treatment they are receiving, because for example placebos are being used, the trial is said to be *blind*.

Third, it is important that the way the outcome of the trial is to be measured is clearly defined. For instance, in a study of neural-tube defects, one must specify exactly which deformities will count as neural-tube defects. This specification is very important. Most trials are carried out by more than one investigator, and it is essential that they are all measuring exactly the same things. Users of the trial results may also need to know exactly what was measured to understand what is going on. (This does not mean that nothing else is ever recorded. For example, if a new drug produces severe, adverse effects in some patients, this would no doubt also be recorded.)

Consider another feature of intervention trial design. Suppose a new drug for treating depression is being tested in a trial, against an old drug. A doctor is asked to report on how patients respond to the drugs. Suppose the doctor knows which patients had which drug. Consciously or unconsciously, this could affect their assessment of the patients' condition, so that any observed difference might again be partly or entirely caused by differences in what is reported rather than real differences between the treatments. To guard against this, the investigators who measure the outcome of the treatment are often kept in the dark about exactly which treatment each patient has received. If the patients are also unaware which treatment

they are receiving, because for example the control group are taking placebos, or new and old drugs are packaged identically, the trial is *double-blind*. Double-blind trials are sound practice because they help to ensure that experimental and control groups are treated alike. But they are not always possible. For instance, in the follow-up to a surgical operation it may be obvious to the observer whether or not a particular procedure has been performed.

The final method of ensuring that experimental and control groups are as similar as possible that we shall discuss is in some ways the most important. Suppose you were running a trial of folic acid to prevent the recurrence of neural-tube defects, and had found a reasonable number of eligible women willing to take part. The control group is to be given placebos.

☐ How would you decide who gets the folic acid and who does not? (Remember that the aim is to make the experimental and control groups as alike as possible.)

■ Perhaps the first thing you would think of doing is to make sure that the age distribution, social class distribution, and so on, are similar in both groups. But the difficulty is the 'and so on'. If you tried to match up the groups like this, there would always be the possibility that you would fail to match them on some important characteristic which you did not even know to be relevant. Instead, the answer would be to allocate the women to the two groups *at random*. For instance, you could toss a coin for each woman. If it was a head, she would get folic acid, if a tail, the placebo.

In practice, this *randomisation* is not usually done by tossing a coin; there are more sophisticated methods, but the principle is the same.

It may seem paradoxical to use a random method, involving chance, to achieve two comparable groups. But a random allocation will tend to achieve roughly the same distribution of age, social class, and anything else you might *or might not* have thought of, in both groups. Much the same reasoning lies behind the use of random samples in surveys. However hard you try to make your sample representative of the population, if random methods are not used the sample might end up being unrepresentative in some way you have not even thought of.

In the folic acid trial, then, if the groups are chosen at random, and if they are sufficiently large, it is unlikely that they will differ systematically except that one gets folic acid and the other does not. This makes it much more plausible that any observed difference in the number of neural-tube defects between the two groups is caused by the folic acid rather than anything else. Randomisation is perhaps the most important feature of a properly run intervention trial; it is the randomisation that enables causal conclusions to be drawn from the results.

However much effort is put into ensuring that the different individuals in the trial are treated in the same way, different people will respond differently to the same treatment. Because individuals vary, and therefore the results of interventions vary from one person to another, statistical techniques such as significance tests are used widely in intervention trials to determine what conclusions can be drawn from the trial results about the general effectiveness of the interventions being studied. So, significance tests and confidence intervals are important in this context. Yet these statistical methods can play an important role even before a trial has started, in helping to determine how many people should be studied.

Obviously, the more individuals that are studied in a trial, the clearer will be the picture given by the results. But there are limitations on the number of people that can be involved. In practical terms, suitable individuals may be hard to find, and resources of time, money and people to conduct the trial are limited. In ethical terms, it is unsatisfactory to conduct a trial after one treatment has been clearly shown to be better, because this would not be in the best interests of the people receiving the inferior treatment. So ideally a trial should include as many individuals as is necessary to judge whether the interventions being studied do really differ to an extent that is medically important, but should not include *more* people than this. Statistical calculations based on the ideas of significance testing can give a firm indication before the trial starts of how many people need to be included to satisfy these objectives, and indeed to determine if a particular trial is worth doing at all. Deciding on the number of people to include in a trial is, or should be, one of the most important parts of its design. A trial that is too small to produce usable results is a waste of resources — and yet such trials have been conducted all too often.

Let us return to the question of providing extra vitamins to women to prevent the recurrence of neural-tube defects. In Part 3 of the Course Reader* there are brief reports of two different trials which investigated the effectiveness of such interventions around the time of conception. The first of these trials is described in Smithells *et al.* (1980) 'Possible prevention of neural-tube defects by periconceptional vitamin supplementation' (Section 3.6). Read the article and the accompanying correspondence from *The Lancet*, and then work through the questions and answers here.

☐ The trial reported by Smithells *et al.* used a group-comparative design. Were women allocated to the groups at random?
■ No. The controls were women who were already

*Black, Nick *et al.* (eds) (1984) *Health and Disease: A Reader*, Open University Press.

pregnant when they entered the study, or who refused the vitamin supplement. In a sense, they mostly chose themselves.
☐ Was the study double-blind?
■ No. The women knew whether or not they were taking vitamins, and so did the investigators.
☐ Briefly summarise the results.
■ Neural-tube defects recurred much less often when mothers had received the vitamin supplement. The difference was statistically significant.
☐ How do the authors interpret this?
■ In the 'Discussion' they put forward four possible interpretations. One is that the vitamin supplementation tends to prevent neural-tube defects, although they noted that this might be a placebo effect. The other explanations are essentially that, for some reason, the groups differed in some way that had nothing to do with the vitamin supplements.

You might have wondered why Professor Smithells and his colleagues did not carry out a double-blind trial using random allocation and placebos. The correspondence shows that they wanted to, but they were not allowed to by some of the ethics committees involved. Research on human subjects in hospitals in Britain has to be approved by such committees, whose function is essentially to make ethical judgements on proposals for research.

A double-blind, randomised trial of folic acid supplementation to prevent the recurrence of neural-tube defects *has* been carried out in Britain, by Laurence and his co-workers in South Wales. Now read the article, 'Double-blind randomised controlled trial of folate treatment before conception to prevent recurrence of neural-tube defects' (Section 3.6), by Laurence *et al.* (1981) in Part 3 of the Course Reader, and then return to the questions here.

☐ In the study by Professor Laurence and his co-workers, out of the 60 pregnancies in women given folate tablets to provide folic acid, there were 2 neural-tube defects. Out of the 51 pregnancies in women given placebos, 4 resulted in neural-tube defects. This difference is not statistically significant. On what basis do Laurence *et al.* argue that folic acid supplementation does work?
■ Essentially, they divided the folic acid group into 'compliers' who had taken the tablets and 'non-compliers' who had not. They did this on the basis of the amount of folate in the bloodstream (in fact, their basis for deciding who complied has been criticised). They then counted the non-compliers in with those who had been given no folic acid to begin with, and there *was* a statistically significant difference ($P = 0.04$) in the recurrence of neural-tube defects between this group and the compliers.

The division of the experimental group into compliers and non-compliers was not done at random; these subgroups were self-selected. But still it could be argued that this study suggested that *folic acid* was effective in reducing the chance of recurrence of neural-tube defects, but that the *intervention* of giving folic acid tablets was not necessarily effective, because the difference between the group given tablets and the group given placebos was not significant.

    ☐   Does this last result mean that giving folic acid tablets has *no* effect on neural-tube defects?

    ■   No. Remember that 'difference not significant' means 'chance not ruled out' — and *that* could be because insufficient evidence was collected. On balance, it may be more likely that the number of individuals in the trial was not large enough to detect a true difference than that the difference really does not exist. But the trial itself is inconclusive on this question.

These two studies, other studies by the same workers and, in particular, the proposal in 1982 to run a further large intervention trial under the auspices of the Medical Research Council*, raised a considerable furore, which spilled out of medical circles into the general press. Questions of ethics in intervention trials became, briefly, a matter of public debate. Some of this controversy is represented by the rest of the material reprinted under the heading, 'Ethical dilemmas in evaluation' (Section 3.6), in the Course Reader. You might like to look at this now if you have time.

    Intervention trials play a major part in medical research. But for various reasons they are more widely used in some areas of medicine than in others. For example, clinical trials are routinely used in drug therapy. (A *clinical trial* is an intervention trial in which the people being studied are patients.) Properly conducted clinical trials of some other types of intervention, such as surgery, are much less common.

* The trial is taking place as we write (1984).

Objectives for Chapter 6

When you have studied this chapter, you should be able to:

    6.1 Define the notions of prospective, retrospective, case-control and cohort studies; distinguish between them, and interpret simple conclusions from such studies.

    6.2 Give examples of the limitations of prospective, retrospective, case-control and cohort studies, and of such observational studies in general.

    6.3 Describe the basic approach of statistical significance testing; interpret conclusions from such tests; and outline the basic limitations of significance testing.

    6.4 Describe the basic methodology of intervention trials and their role in identifying causes. Define the terms 'control group' and 'placebo'.

    6.5 Justify the role of a double-blind design and randomisation in intervention trials; explain why it is important to specify criteria for selecting people to take part, to specify the treatments exactly and to define how the outcome will be measured.

Questions for Chapter 6

1 (*Objectives 6.1 and 6.2*) (a) In 1939, F. H. Müller reported the results of an investigation of lung cancer and smoking. He studied a group of people with lung cancer, and another matched group who did not have the disease. He found that the cancer patients had smoked much more than the people in the other group. Was this a retrospective or a prospective study? Was it a case-control or a cohort study?

    (b) In 1956, Richard Doll and A. Bradford Hill published the first main report on their findings from a prospective cohort study in which they sent questionnaires to all male British doctors about their smoking habits, and recorded lung cancer deaths among the doctors as they occurred. They reported that the age-standardised death rate from lung cancer among doctors who were heavy smokers was 166 per hundred thousand, and that this was 24 times the rate of 7 per hundred thousand for non-smoking doctors. Could death rates such as these be calculated from the results of a case-control study?

2 (*Objectives 6.3–6.5*) Multiple sclerosis is a chronic degenerative disease of the nervous system for which there is at present (1984) no known cure. Suppose you discover a drug which, on the basis of animal trials and some preliminary tests on humans, seems as if it might have a beneficial effect on multiple sclerosis patients. The drug is taken in tablet form. You decide to carry out a group comparative trial of the new drug.

(a) One group will receive the new drug. What treatment will the other group receive?

(b) You have available a number of patients who satisfy the eligibility criteria for the trial and have consented to take part. How do you decide which patients receive the treatment?

(c) After the patients have had the course of treatment, a doctor will assess their condition. Should he or she know which treatment each patient has been given?

(d) Suppose the doctor rates each patient's condition on a scale from 0 (no symptoms) to 4 (very severely ill). A statistical significance test is to be carried out to investigate whether your new drug has an effect. Say (in words) what the null hypothesis would be.

(e) The difference between the two groups turns out to be 'not statistically significant'. Does this mean that your drug has no effect at all?

7

Human social organisation

The principal aim of Chapters 7–11 is to introduce you to the range of methods that social scientists use, and to get you to think generally about the problems of human social behaviour. You are not expected to learn how to use these methods, nor to remember *all* the technical terms. The main point is to develop a critical approach to social science data.

Social science, like natural science, has its origins in the sixteenth and seventeenth centuries. In most of its disciplines, however, and unlike biology, health and disease were for a long time only marginal topics for investigation. Outside psychology (the study of individuals) and demography (the study of populations) such matters were left largely to doctors, and they in their turn focused mostly upon biology. The result of this mutual neglect, if we turn again to diabetes, is that a good deal less is known on the social side.

Why should this be important? Diabetes, like every disease, can be investigated in several ways. We can look at its manifestation in the body of the individual — the approach of the clinician and the biologist. Or, we can examine its distribution across large numbers of people — the approach of the epidemiologist. However, what is still missing is a specifically *social* investigation.

□   What do we mean by 'social'? Think about its definition for a moment. You might also look it up in a dictionary.

■   Your dictionary may have said something like this: '1. *a*. Living in companies or organized communities, gregarious ...; not fitted for or not practising solitary life; interdependent, co-operative, practising division of labour, existing only as member of compound organism, (of insects) having common nests etc., (of birds) building near each other in communities; (of plants) growing thickly together and monopolizing ground they grow on. 2. Concerned with the mutual relations of (classes of) human beings ....' (*The Concise Oxford Dictionary*, 6th edn)

□   So what is the difference between the way epidemiologists and social scientists approach diabetes?

■ Social scientists view human beings as far more than individuals, whether considered separately or aggregated. To the social scientist, human beings cannot be understood outside their *relationships* with other human beings. Social science is thus the study of these relationships as much as of the individuals themselves.

'Social' is a word that we can use right across the biological realm. It does not apply solely to human beings. However, although many other species are gregarious, live in communities or have relationships with one another, the complexity and variety of human social relationships has no parallel in the rest of the biological realm.

Why should this be so? Consider first one of the simplest forms of life, the amoeba, and one of the simplest forms of relationship — that existing between a single amoeba and its environment. This is not a social relationship according to the dictionary definition. We need another amoeba for that. And yet, on closer inspection, a primitive form of sociality is involved. We cannot understand the amoeba just by itself; it is in constant interaction with the world around it.

Put a single amoeba or bacterium in a glass of water with a drop of sugar solution at one side of it. The organism will move towards the sugar solution, from an environment without sugar to one that is sugar-rich; it will *select* its environment. Once there, it will absorb the sugar, convert it metabolically into a variety of products and spit them out again. It will thus take part of its environment into itself, and transform it into more of itself. At the same time it will actively transform its environment, which will change as a result of its being there. As a result of that change the environment itself may become less favourable to the organism; it may turn more acid, for example. The organism will then move out of that environment to another, more favourable one. This simple organism is actively transforming its environment.

Now compare amoebae with human beings. Humans too select and modify their environments, but they can do these things in a far more powerful way than amoebae, because they can also *reflect* in enormous detail upon themselves, their choices and their environments, both natural and social. This capacity for reflection is given by language and is the reason why humans, more than any other species, can re-make both the natural and their own social world. It is also, to give a more trivial example, the basis of this text. Language enables humans to teach and to learn, and it permits them to collaborate in novel and complex projects in ways that other species cannot, however gregarious they might be.

So human social life is extraordinarily complex and varied. However, it is possible to view it, at the very simplest, as consisting of three separate but interdependent levels; that of the *individual*, that of *direct interaction between individuals* and that of *groups*. (The group level is made up of both direct and *indirect* interactions.) At first sight, it might seem that only the last two levels are truly social.

□ Can you think of any reasons why the individual level also involves the social?

■ Individuals think about, react to and act upon the wider social levels, and they are shaped by the kinds of interactions and groups of which they are a part.

Consider the effects and causes of disease at each of these three levels.

The individual

□ What are some possible causes of disease at the individual level?

■ You may have considered matters such as character, the way individuals handle emotions and cope with stress, and the sorts of stress they are exposed to.

The physician, Thomas Willis wrote of diabetes in 1684, 'Sadness or long sorrow, as likewise convulsions and other depressions and disorders of the animal spirits are used to generate or foment this morbid condition' (quoted in Wilkinson, 1981, p.1). However, despite the frequency with which such assertions about diabetes have been made over the centuries, and despite the fact that personality and stress play a part in the causation of some conditions, with diabetes, so far at least, scientists have drawn a blank. This is not true, however, of the effect of diabetes upon the life of the individual diabetic.

□ List the sorts of impact that disease may have upon an individual's life.

■ Physical or mental impairments can affect people in a very large number of ways: disease can limit or modify the range of normal activities, as can its treatment; acute attacks of illness may remove an individual from ordinary life entirely; treatment may require careful monitoring by the patient, by relatives or by medical personnel; both treatment and impairment may render the individual dependent on others; the individual may actively be barred from certain occupations or activities; many conditions pose the threat of death much more vividly; disease renders people abnormally conscious of their physical or mental condition; many sufferers are stigmatised by others; disease may be a regular source of pain or anxiety, which may in turn affect relations with others.

This is a very wide range of effects. Many diseases have only a few. But diabetes can illustrate every one of these categories, though fortunately not every diabetic is so affected. Still, it strikes hard. Two psychiatrists, R. B. Tattersall and J. G. L. Jackson, noted in a recent review:

> The newly diagnosed diabetic is confronted by a new vocabulary, a need to learn food values previously ignored, a new responsibility for administering his own treatment, the frightening immediate or remote possibility of self-injection and anxiety about the possibility of hypoglycaemia (a word which he probably does not understand anyway) and apparently terrifying medical complications.... Diet enforces the greatest change in life-style. Food has a deep psychological significance as a biological sign of love and affection, a source of oral gratification and a comfort in anxiety-producing situations ... [note that] companion means literally 'one with whom one takes bread' .... (Tattersall and Jackson, 1982, p.272)

Given this, what is striking about the impact of diabetes is how well most diabetics cope with it. For example, a range of studies has shown that mental disorder is no more common among diabetics than among the rest of the population. Human beings are clearly tough and flexible, able to cope with quite dramatic changes in their personal circumstances. There is, however, likely to be quite a lengthy period of adjustment. Getting used to any radical change in one's life takes time. Moreover, research also suggests that although diabetics are no more likely than anyone else to be 'disturbed', those who are (particularly children) are liable to be more so. An editorial in the medical journal, *The Lancet*, suggests some of the reasons why:

> The need for discipline in diet, urine testing and insulin administration, and the alarming consequences of rule-breaking, not only provide ample opportunity for confrontation between child, parent and doctor, but also place a set of trump cards in the hands of a manipulative youngster. (*The Lancet*, 1980, p.189)

□ This quotation illustrates at least three further features of the impact of illness upon the individual. What are they?
■ Illness can sometimes be used as an *excuse*; it is therefore subject to *moral judgement*; and its treatment renders the individual the object of *control* by others.

Excuses, control and moral judgement all, in their different ways, point to wider social features, beyond the individual. It is time to consider the next level of social organisation.

Direct interaction

Just as each person, in a limited sense, constitutes a little world of their own, so another little world is formed when two or more people interact with one another, on the street, in meetings, in conversation or on the phone. Each such occasion has its own set of *rules* governing polite behaviour and an array of *roles* appropriate to the various participants. Such rules only regulate outward behaviour; covertly, people may be doing and thinking all kinds of things at variance with their official roles. An important part of human society is constructed out of these innumerable meetings and conversations; or, to use a technical term, from *encounters*.

Most of the time such encounters run fairly smoothly, with not too much discrepancy between overt roles and what is being done covertly. This is, however, not always so. Most diabetics adjust to their lot and therefore most consultations with medical staff go relatively smoothly. However, it is hard for some diabetics to achieve good control of their blood sugar level. When things go wrong, is it because such control is physically impossible or is it because the patient has been lax? How can the dietitian or the doctor tell? It is possible for medical staff's overt attempts to help the patient to turn into covert moral judgements which may threaten the whole relationship. In extreme instances, as two psychiatrists, M. Fabrykant and B. L. Pacella, noted nearly forty years ago, the following may result:

> The patients are anxious to keep sugar-free but dread the incapacitating reactions. If they remain sugar-free through the excessive use of insulin, they develop a constant state of hypoglycaemic anxiety [a physical state], which is often mistaken for psychoneurosis, hysteria, etc. If, on the other hand, glycosuria [excess sugar in the urine] cannot be avoided, they live in fear of diabetic complications and are apt to develop a feeling of guilt. Suspected then by their physicians of breaking the diet and lack of honesty, or stigmatized as neurotics and hypochondriacs, they feel humiliated and lose faith in the medical profession. (quoted in Tattersall and Jackson, 1982, p.275)

Such problems are not unique to the medical world. Similar disturbances may sometimes occur in other encounters. Husband may fall out with wife, parent with child.

The group

□ Human beings belong to innumerable 'groups' with which individuals interact either directly or indirectly. List some of the main social groups to which Mr Lawson 'belongs' or which might influence his diabetes and the treatment for his condition.

■ His family, his friends, those he works with, the medical professions, the businesses that manufacture diabetic foods and drugs will all have an effect. More widely, there are his social class, his gender, his education, his religion, his age, his language, his nationality and his ethnicity.

Let us consider just two of these complex relationships. Take the impact of diabetes on the family of the diabetic. Not much is known about the impact of Type II (maturity-onset) diabetes. However, a good deal of work has been done on the impact of Type I (juvenile-onset). For example, one study compared the mental state of mothers of diabetic children with that of another group of mothers who were similar in many characteristics but whose children were not diabetic. Twenty-eight per cent of the mothers of diabetic children but only 11 per cent of the others in the control group were found to be 'mentally disturbed', a difference largely resulting from the much greater level of anxiety among the mothers of diabetic children. Not surprisingly, some mothers of diabetic children seem to become intensely anxious, sometimes obsessively so. This might appear, at first sight, to be an effect that operates purely at the individual level; but because individuals make up groups, it also has a group effect. The whole family is likely to be influenced in one way or another.

Now consider how social class affects diabetes.

☐ Research has shown a link between nutrition and Type II diabetes. How might social class be involved?
■ People from different social classes, given their different incomes and culture, eat different sorts of food. Those in a 'lower' social class are particularly likely to be obese and thus more vulnerable to Type II diabetes. (This hypothesis was confirmed by an American study that found rates of diabetes to be substantially higher among lower income groups.)

Social class also affects the kinds of resources that patients bring to their struggle with the disease. If, for example, Mr Lawson is forced to retire early because of his diabetes, as a plumber he is likely to receive a smaller pension than someone from a 'higher' social class. In addition, diabetics are particularly vulnerable to the effects of cigarette smoking on the blood vessels, and smoking is, at least nowadays, strongly associated with social class. The 'lower' Mr Lawson's social class, the more likely he is to smoke.

Having reviewed the three levels of social life, let us think once again about their nature and interrelationships. First, note that each level involves the others. Interaction is conducted by individuals, groups have individual members, and so on. Note also that so far we have given detailed consideration to only one type of interaction — that occurring directly between individuals. There is, however, the realm of *indirect interaction* which combines with the direct form to make up the group level. Consider, for example, the transactions, trading, exchanges and markets through which material life is conducted. Direct encounters play a part in this sphere of human activity, but individuals and groups also interact in indirect but profoundly important ways. Though they may never meet, the lives of Mr Lawson, of a Brazilian sugar plantation worker, and of a North American office worker (and the health of all three of them) are shaped by the powerful sinews of economic exchange.

Thus when social scientists talk of 'groups' (or 'institutions' or 'systems' or 'structures') they mean something more than the 'group' of people sitting in out-patients, or the meeting of a local branch of the diabetics association, for example. 'Groups', used in this wider sense, refers to people whom most members of that group may never see and to whom they may feel no sense of belonging and yet with whom they are linked by their common situation or place in a chain of transactions.

Objectives for Chapter 7

When you have studied this chapter, you should be able to:

7.1 Describe how social science is the study of social relationships.

7.2 Outline the three principal levels of social organisation: individual, direct interaction and group (group also involves indirect interaction).

Questions for Chapter 7

1 (*Objective 7.1*) In what way is epidemiology, the study of the distribution of disease within a population, not a fully social science?

2 (*Objective 7.2*) 'That doctor becomes anxious every time she sees Mr Lawson.' What levels of social organisation are referred to in this statement?

3 (*Objective 7.2*) 'So I went and got some tablets from the chemist.' Look at the types of interaction implied by this statement and describe them. Are they direct or indirect?

8
The methodology of social science

Mr Lawson's social class, his family life and the kind of relationship he has with his dietitian can all affect his diabetes. Suppose you wanted to conduct a study of this. How would you go about it? In particular, what sorts of methods should you choose? The study of the reasons why it is better to choose one method rather than another is known as *methodology*. The methodology of social science is rather different from that of biology, epidemiology or clinical medicine.

☐ What were the principal methods used by the biological sciences described in Chapter 3 of this book?
■ At least four significant methods were mentioned: experimentation, animal models, measurement and observation.

Experimentation

Experimentation is the favoured method of proof in the natural sciences. There are several difficulties with experimentation on human *social* behaviour. Some key aspects of human behaviour are impossible to subject to experimental control: they are too complex, or else bedevilled by time. To control a whole society, or to experiment with the past is beyond our power. There are also matters in which control is technically feasible, but politically or ethically impossible. Last, there is the unusual character of human consciousness. Human behaviour can change dramatically if people know they are being experimented upon.

The first problem, the impossibility of controlling some aspects of social life, has counterparts in the study of evolution and ethology (the investigation of the social behaviour of animals). But the others are special. Consider first the human reaction to being experimented with. This is often known as the 'Hawthorne effect' from some famous experiments carried out in an electrical component factory of that name in the 1930s. Researchers were hired to find ways of increasing the productivity of the plant. They were given *carte blanche* to modify the physical environment, the way the workers were treated, and the manner in which they were paid. After a bit, they noticed something rather odd. Whatever they did, productivity kept on rising. Even changes that might have been expected to lower production had the opposite effect.

☐ What might explain this continuing rise in productivity?
■ The researchers eventually concluded that because the work was so boring, the workers were rather pleased with the interest they were getting from the researchers. What they were responding to was simply the fact that they were being experimented upon. It was this, not the content of any particular experiment, that was having the effect.

Since the American psychologists Roethlisberger and Dickson carried out this work, other psychologists have gone to highly ingenious lengths to design experiments that would limit the Hawthorne effect. There has been some success. Nevertheless, the ghost of the Hawthorne study still haunts social science; experimentation is mostly confined to a single discipline, that of psychology, where it can focus on individuals and immediate effects, and where there is some possibility of tight control.

Given these various problems, experimentation will never occupy as dominant a position in the social sciences as it does in biology and medicine. However, more might be done. When the clinical trial was first introduced, many doctors held that medical practice was too complex for the experimental method. It might work in agricultural research where the randomised trial was first developed, but medicine was an art as much as a science. This attitude has largely faded over the past thirty years. Yet the application of the clinical trial to areas of life beyond medicine meets the fierce resistance that doctors once used to offer. Many social workers, for example, see trials as unethical and are unwilling to let therapy be randomised. yet it seems possible that clinical trials will prove of major benefit to social work practice also.

There may also be scope for a greater use of less rigorous experimentation. There are some fascinating American experiments in which researchers have posed as mental patients to study aspects of psychiatric diagnosis. This form of research could well be extended. The experimental method could also be applied more systematically to the running of different types of organisations. This is already done to a limited extent. Aside from 'action research' there are 'pilot' projects, 'experimental units', and so forth. However, much of our society operates with a very limited time span and expects instant 'solutions' to problems. This attitude is not compatible with long-term organisational experimentation.

Animal models

Biologists, faced with difficulties in human experimentation turn to animals. Should social scientists do the same? There have been several popular attempts to do this recently, including Desmond Morris's work, *The Naked Ape*, the various books of Robert Ardrey and the 'sociobiology' of E. O. Wilson, a Harvard entomologist. (Entomology is the study of insects, and Wilson first made his name in the study of insect societies.) There are two grave difficulties with such an approach. First, the behaviour of every species is different. Even arguing from one type of rat to another can present problems. Second, because of the existence of human language, our social behaviour is far more complex and varied than that of other species.

Studies comparing humans and animals must therefore be approached with great caution. There is likely to be something that we can learn about ourselves by studying other species, and biologists often borrow models of human society and apply them to other species. However, the comparison is a difficult one in our present state of knowledge. Social scientists are largely ignorant of ethology, the science of animal social behaviour, and ethology itself is relatively new and underdeveloped. Much of our social knowledge of animals still comes from the study of the captive and specially bred, and is therefore of uncertain relevance. In the future, perhaps, social scientists may use 'ethological plausibility' as a criterion for discussing the merits of a new hypothesis. For the time being, the comparative study of human social life looks merely to history and to anthropology, to other human beings in other times and places.

Observation

Experimentation and animal models do not work very well in the study of human social behaviour. *Observation* fortunately does. It does not, however, work in quite the same fashion as in the natural sciences.

☐ What special features occur to you about the role of observation in the human social sciences? (Think particularly about the possession of language and just who is being studied.)

■ First, because they are studying themselves people are liable to be biased and to have special insiders' knowledge. Second, given their possession of language and a capacity for reflection, all humans are social observers, and because the social world is so important to them humans are quite good at certain sorts of observation. This has two consequences: (a) professional social scientists face serious amateur competition, but (b) at the same time they can enlist their subjects' aid in a way that natural scientists cannot.

Some of these points may need elaboration. Take first the argument that everyone is a social observer. Everyone observes the natural world. Yet few, nowadays, except gamekeepers or bird-watchers, have any detailed knowledge of that world. Amateurs rarely pose any serious threat to the professionals. This was not always so: tribal people's knowledge of the natural world is most elaborate, and natural science was once a gentleman's hobby. King Charles II was a founder of the leading British scientific society, 'The Royal Society' (hence its name). In the nineteenth century amateurs had a major role in the discovery of new species; now they are a rare species themselves. However, it seems unlikely that humans will ever lose their detailed knowledge of the social world. Watching people and studying the way organisations work have a special importance. Without a certain minimum competence in these matters, it would be hard to get through life at all.

The status of professional social scientists is therefore lower than that of natural scientists, and likely to remain so. One of the big advantages of physics is that electrons cannot answer back. However wrong the physicist's analysis, however partial and simple-minded, the only source of criticism is other physicists, who may all share their colleague's naïvety or prejudices. Social scientists, by contrast, face keen competition. For example, there are the subjects of their research and those who sponsor it. Sometimes they may like it, but they may also say that it is banal, that they knew it already, or that it is plain wrong. Besides social scientists, there is a galaxy of other professional observers who also make their livings from studying the social world — novelists, journalists, film-makers and dramatists, politicians and policemen.

Whatever the disadvantages for the status of the social scientist, such competition does help humanity's chances of understanding its social life. Compared with the biological sciences, social science can begin from a detailed knowledge base, and the presence of so many other competent practitioners means that theories and findings are potentially subject to a greater range of informed criticism. Moreover, rather than seeing other social observers as merely competitors, social scientists can enlist their aid. Many social science data are therefore 'secondary' for they consist of the research subject's own observations of the social world. Finally, methods and theories too can be borrowed. Very few social theories are likely to be entirely original.

☐ If everyone is, in a sense, a social scientist, what can professionals do that others do not?

■ Everyone observes their own social world, but this is normally a sideline, subordinate to some more immediate, practical task. Social scientists have no need to be as hasty as journalists, as dependent on popular taste as film-makers, or as partial as the Special Branch.

This distinctive relationship to the social world has three important consequences. It enables data to be collected more systematically. It permits a more focused testing of different theories. (Everyone can produce a plausible explanation — or several — and therein lies the snag. Social scientists have the time to explore the implications of each theory and to check these against the data.) Finally, it enables the professional to study things that are too removed from the amateur's immediate concerns to receive much serious attention.

Measurement

Measurement too takes a different form in social sciences.

☐ Imagine that Mr Lawson is dissatisfied with his doctor, worried that he really has cancer, and decides to pay for a private consultation. What sorts of things might be readily measured in these circumstances, and what other things might prove harder to quantify?

■ It is easy to count the consultation time and the fee, and to note the gender and age of both Mr Lawson and the doctor. But what about their social class, emotions and actions and the wider costs such meetings create?

Plumbing is a skilled occupation and often quite well-paid. Does Mr Lawson have rather more in common with those in many middle-class occupations than he does with, say, an unskilled labourer? Moreover, people differ in the way they define social class: some deny the reality of class; others think it is the only important thing in life. Quantifying the evaluation of emotion or experience is also tricky. 'It was all right really' makes sense but is difficult to measure. Was it really all right or was it unpleasant? And if it was in fact unpleasant, precisely how unpleasant? These questions are hard to answer, for under inspection, good things have their bad sides too; every silver lining has a cloud. There are also problems in classifying actions. Did the doctor give Mr Lawson a real welcome, did she treat him with some deference, or was she merely polite? These are delicate matters of judgement. Finally, what was the wider emotional cost of seeing this doctor in these circumstances?

None of these problems of classification and quantification is completely insuperable. Measurement has a major role in the social sciences. However, because of the complexity and variety of human society, purely descriptive, non-numerical methods, have an important part to play.

☐ Where have you come across non-numerical methods before in the study of health and disease?

■ The clinical method is non-numerical, or *qualitative* not quantitative.

Qualitative methods are also used in some areas of biology such as ethology. However, with these few exceptions, biomedical research is dominated by numerical methods, and much of the success of scientific medicine is based on increasing quantification. Social science (so far at least) is different: qualitative methods are still the dominant form in certain disciplines, particularly history and anthropology, and are of considerable importance in both sociology and politics. Numerical methods predominate in demography, economics, geography and psychology. Much of the earlier part of this book has been devoted to numerical methods; it is time to give qualitative techniques a closer look.

Objective for Chapter 8

When you have studied this chapter, you should be able to:

8.1 Describe the principal methods of the social sciences and state how and why these differ from those of natural science.

Question for Chapter 8

1 (*Objective 8.1*) Different surgeons have different criteria for when to perform a hysterectomy. This may be the result of the training they receive in different medical schools. To test this hypothesis, you might think of doing the following: (i) chatting to them about it; (ii) making videotapes of surgeons being trained; (iii) checking to see if there is any association between surgeons' criteria for performing surgery and the particular medical school they attended; (iv) modifying the training in selected medical schools and seeing what happens; (v) varying the conditions under which a group of chimpanzees live to see how this affects the way they help each other when they are ill.

(a) Which of the following methods — experiment, animal modelling and observation — would be used in each of (i)–(v)?

(b) In which of (i)–(v) could we use accurate measurement? In which might this be difficult?

(c) What are the advantages and disadvantages of each method in testing the hypothesis? Which method would you choose?

9
Qualitative methods

This chapter contains references to the Course Reader, so have it by you as you work. You will be asked to read the extract by Jan van den Berg (1981), reprinted in Part 6, Section 6.1. You are not obliged to read the other extract we mention (Posner, 1977, reprinted in Part I, Section 1.7), but it is interesting background reading if you have time.

Her throat was contracting into hollows with each breath, her veins were swollen and her face was turning from pink to a pale lilac. I immediately realized what this colouring meant. I made my first diagnosis which was not only correct but, more importantly, was given at the same moment as the midwives with all their experience.

'The little girl has diphtherial croup. Her throat is already choked with membrane and soon it will be blocked completely.'

'How long has she been ill?' I asked, breaking the tense silence of my assistants.

'Five days now,' the mother answered, staring hard at me with dry eyes.

'Diphtheria,' I said to the *feldsher* through clenched teeth and turned to the mother: 'Why have you left it so long?'

At that moment I heard a tearful voice behind me: 'Five days Sir, five days!' I turned round and saw that a round-faced old woman had silently come in. 'I wish these old women didn't exist,' I thought to myself. With an aching presentiment of trouble I said: 'Quiet, woman, you're only in the way' and repeated to the mother: 'Why have you left it so long? Five days? Hmm?'

Suddenly with an automatic movement the mother handed the little girl to the grandmother and sank to her knees in front of me.

'Give her some medicine,' she said and banged her forehead on the floor. 'I'll kill myself if she dies.'

'Get up at once,' I replied, 'Or I won't even talk to you.'
(Bulgakov, 1975, pp.31–2)

This is from a short story first published in 1927 by the Russian novelist Mikhail Bulgakov. It is a work of fiction. Before becoming a writer, Bulgakov had been a doctor, practising at first in a remote part of Russia where the people had their own medical beliefs and distrusted modern Western medicine.

☐ What do we normally mean by calling something 'fiction'?

■ The *Concise Oxford Dictionary* says: 'Feigning, invention, invented statement or narrative; literature consisting of such narrative; conventionally accepted falsehood (especially legal or polite fiction).'

This is a literal definition. It hardly does justice to Bulgakov, or to many other works of fiction. It is instead more accurate to see fiction as a convention which grants writers a licence to make things up and offers a defence against possible libel. But writers can still use the convention to engage in detailed social analysis.

☐ What advantages might fiction have over other forms of analysis?

■ Two advantages may have come to mind, the first to do with the necessity to entertain, the second to do with the difficulties of access to particular topics.

Some of our best portraits of medicine and of sickness come from the writers of fiction. Many writers first trained as doctors: Tobias Smollett in the eighteenth century; Anton Chekhov in the nineteenth century; and, in this century, A. J. Cronin, Somerset Maugham, Louis-Ferdinand Céline in France, and Arthur Schnitzler in Vienna; not forgetting three recent satirists of contemporary medical life, Richard Gordon, Colin Douglas and Samuel Shem (author of *House of God*, the *Catch-22* of the American hospital). Lay views of health and disease are too numerous to list, but good examples are George Eliot's *Middlemarch*, Simone de Beauvoir's *A Very Easy Death* and Peter Nicholl's two plays, *The National Health* and *A Day in the Death of Joe Egg*. Even television soap-operas such as *Angels* can be valuable.

Introspection

Bulgakov's story is unusual and dramatic, yet novelty and drama are relatively infrequent occurrences in everyday life. Most of our days are spent in routines that we take for granted and therefore fail to analyse. Many of these routines are important for students of health and disease. How should they be studied? Turn to the extract, 'The meaning of being ill', by Jan van den Berg (1981) in the Course Reader (Part 6, Section 6.1), and study it carefully.

☐ How does van den Berg manage to study things that are normally taken for granted?

■ Van den Berg uses the unusual, the acute illness, to reveal aspects of the everyday world that normally pass unnoticed. He then uses what he has discovered about the usual to analyse the unusual further.

Van den Berg is a student of *phenomenology*, the study of how people experience the world introspectively. It is

harder to do this systematically than it looks. For much of their lives people fly on auto-pilot: they get by through sets of routines, concentrating only on the novel and immediately problematic. Social scientists too can neglect everyday aspects, unless they take particular care.

☐ Bulgakov and van den Berg based their analyses on the observation of their own lives. What problems might there be in studying your life *solely* through this method?

■ How adequate is your own sampling of social life? How biased is your interpretation of what you can see?

Even when people do notice things they are liable to be biased by their personal interests. Their focus is always selective and their memory fallible. Moreover, because human societies are as varied as human lives, what one person sees is a tiny fraction of the whole. Just as many aspects of the body's interior are hidden and require X-rays and biochemical tests for their investigation, so students of social life need additional methods to study those parts that everyday observation cannot reach!

Participant observation

Bulgakov observed the people that he happened to meet. It is, however, possible to try to live another's life for a while. George Orwell became a tramp in order to write *Down and Out in London and Paris*, and the method has been used by writers, journalists and scientists since the nineteenth century. Social scientists usually call it *participant observation*.

☐ What are some of the advantages of participant observation compared with simply observing one's own life?

■ Many more aspects of the 'borrowed' life are likely to appear 'strange' to the participant observer, though routine to those who ordinarily live it. The problem of ignoring the familiar is thereby reduced. Likewise, the outsider will not be subject to the same set of personal interests and biases.

☐ What special disadvantage might this method have?

■ Participant observation works easily only for low-status occupations or in public settings. (It is not difficult to do research on tramps or kitchen-hands by this method, but studying surgeons and Ministers of Health presents problems.)

What effect might the presence of an observing social scientist have? The observer-effect might seem particularly worrying at first. The workers in the Hawthorne plant changed their behaviour because they were being experimented upon; is observation as unreliable as experimentation? Most experiments create an artificial situation, whereas observation does not actively seek to modify what people are doing. In addition, because there are many aspects of human lives of which those who lead them are hardly aware, the presence of an observer may have little effect. Above all, it is remarkable what people will actually permit. Consider the startling things revealed by television documentaries of schools, families and the police!

Non-participant observation

One way round some of these problems is to observe but not participate. Systematic observation began in anthropology around the turn of the century. Up till then it had been an armchair discipline whose data came mainly from missionaries and travellers. The quality of this material was poor, and so anthropologists began instead to spend several years living among the people they wished to study, learning their language and getting to know the culture at first hand. Their success with this method abroad led some to try it at home. Journalists too, had an influence on the method.

Here is a passage from a recent observational study of surgery by Charles Bosk, an American sociologist. ('Attendings' is the name for the senior doctors who practise in the hospital but are not on its staff — a standard feature of American hospitals. Only the trainees, that is, the 'residents' and 'interns' are actually staff members.)

A second common judgemental error of attendings is the failure to establish a clear-cut plan of action for chronic problems. For most of these patients, secondary problems make operating impossible. These patients tend to linger in the hospital. They are not discharged, nor are they aggressively treated. Often diagnostic tests reveal conditions in addition to the original problem requiring hospitalization. Each test in turn requires a further one. Intensive diagnostic studies are done on the patient even though he will not be extensively treated: [Bosk then quotes the Chief Resident] 'Surgeons in general don't like theoretical or psychological problems. Things are either black or white. If they don't understand something, they try to put it out of their minds. For example, there are two patients on our service right now whom we can't do anything with, and they really need something done. I think they will die without operations. But they are too sick to be operated on.... One of the worst things that can happen to a patient is to spend a long time on a surgical service. Surgeons lose interest in chronic problems.... Unfortunately some patients, not a lot, die because the surgeon loses interest.' (Bosk, 1979, p.48)

Note that although this is a piece of qualitative research, it does use primitive forms of counting. The phrases used here, such as 'common', 'most', and 'tend to', are standard in such research. (Qualitative research also uses terms such as 'always', 'rarely', 'only in the following circumstances' and 'never'.) Such terms are also characteristic of lay speech — 'surgeons in general', says the Chief Resident. The author then tries to warrant his analysis by citing a quotation, which illustrates the general thesis he himself has just put forward.

Faction

We began this chapter with an extract from a work of fiction. Now consider the following description.

After the operation the patient continued to be puzzled about why all the doctors had been so evasive about reporting the test results, when doing so would seemingly have assured her that she had a curable disease and would have saved her from two days of extreme distress ... she asked her physician if she could read her chart [case-records] but even after obtaining his permission when she went to the nurses' station and reached out to take the record, a nurse stopped her hand and pushed it away ... the nurse smugly informed her that even though her medical physician had agreed, when her surgeon had been informed of her request to see the chart he had left word that she was not to be allowed to look at it.

... She decided not to raise the matter at first but to await his (the surgeon's) response. He came by moments later, and after silently checking on her wound, he turned to go, having made no reference to his veto of her request. She called to him as he was stepping out the door:

'Dr. Williams — I understand you object to my seeing my chart. Would you mind telling me why?'

He looked unperturbed and replied:

'It's not that I object. But it's not our policy to show our patients their charts. And our patients don't want to see their charts.'

She raised her eyebrows in mock surprise and answered sweetly:

'But I want to see my chart. That's why I asked to see it.'

A smile of contempt crossed his face.

'Why do you want to see your chart? It's really not very interesting reading.'

She replied:

'Because I'd like to know all the facts pertinent to my illness.'

[Eventually, after quite a battle, the surgeon gives her the chart.]

After returning to her room she shut the door behind her and climbed into bed with the chart ... Hurriedly she searched through the record for the report on the liver biopsy. She discovered that it was only a single line written on an otherwise blank sheet of paper. It merely read: 'No analysis, Specimen Insufficient for Diagnosis.' (Millman, 1978, pp.142–4)

This is from a recent study of surgery by the American sociologist, Marcia Millman.

    ☐   Do you have any doubts about its authenticity? List them.
    ■   Several doubts may have occurred to you. How much of this is based upon the author's observation and how much upon the patient's report? How far can we believe everything that people tell us and how far can we be certain that, for example, it really was a 'smile of contempt'? What criteria have we got for recognising such things? And, finally, does not the style of the description seem rather closer to the novel form than to that of social science? (There is a smooth villain, a battling heroine, a surprise ending, and some purple prose.)

How legitimate is it to write social science in the quasi-novel form and to take such apparent liberties with the data? The argument against is that it is unlikely that events happened precisely in this fashion. The vivid style is a deception. The defence is that, given its fictional style, it is not making the same claims to the literal truth that are implicit within a more neutral 'scientific' style. By presenting her findings in a quasi-novel form, the author renders her work easier to read, but pays a price in credibility. The form is a common one nowadays, sometimes termed *faction* to convey its ambiguous status. It is normally used either by investigative journalists, or by novelists who have turned to writing documentary material.

Informal interviewing
Bosk and Millman got their data not just from their own observation of surgery but from the observations made by surgeons and patients. Most social scientists make a sharp distinction between these two sorts of data, often keeping the term 'observation' solely for those they have made themselves. *Other people's* observations on the world are given different names: *interviews*, in the case of spoken reports made directly to the social scientist, *diaries* in the case of reports made directly to themselves, and so on.

    ☐   Does this differ from the use of the term 'observation' in natural science?
    ■   Biologists and epidemiologists see both participant observation *and* interview data as observational data, because both are descriptive and non-experimental.

    ☐   Why might social scientists and natural scientists have come to use this term in different ways?
    ■   Human beings have a monopoly on scientific observation of the natural world — as far as we know! Physicists report on electrons; electrons do not report on them, or on each other. Social scientists have no such monopoly on observation, so they are forced to make a careful distinction between what they themselves observe and what is merely reported to them by others.

Just as one cannot necessarily trust one's own observations, so there are special reasons why interview data should not always be trusted. People may not have any opinions upon a subject until asked about them. Or, they may say what they think the questioner would like to hear. In either instance, the data may be an *artefact*, something that was created by the method of investigation itself. Another danger is that what people *say* and what people *do* are different things. The commonest mistake in research based on interviews is to claim that it reveals people's behaviour directly, when it merely provides subjective and potentially unreliable *reports* on that behaviour. The classic demonstration of this was a study of racial prejudice conducted in the 1930s by Richard LaPiere, an American sociologist (see Deutscher, 1969). The white owners of various restaurants and hotels in the United States were asked whether they would accept Chinese as customers. Many said they would not. Six months earlier and unknown to them, LaPiere had tested their actual response to one of these groups by sending them a Chinese couple as customers. (LaPiere accompanied them most of the time.) The proprietors' actual behaviour did not correspond with what they said. The couple were refused service only once!

LaPiere conducted his interviews by postal questionnaire. He might have got slightly different results if he had asked his questions informally, by chatting to the owners. Informality is the key feature of qualitative interviewing. Ideally, the researcher allows the person they are interviewing to talk at length. There is often no set list of questions, merely a rough set of topics that can be explored as and when seems appropriate. Many qualitative studies rely solely on this method.

Informal interviewing is essentially exploratory. It is ideal for investigating the subtle, the complex and the controversial. Researchers are therefore *not* necessarily looking for the frequency with which things are said. Instead, they are often trying to get people to reveal and reflect more than they might normally do. Here is an example taken from an interview study by the anthropologist Tina Posner of a doctor doing just that. (Extracts from her article, 'Magical elements in orthodox medicine', have been included, as background reading, in Part 1, Section 1.7 of the Course Reader.)

... although evidence is not weighted heavily in favour of good control reducing complications, we all *secretly feel* that this is in fact the case, that if you can control the patient's diabetes as well as possible it *should* retard the development of complications. We all *secretly believe* this and *hope* about it, but there is no outstanding evidence that it is true. There have been a number of papers that support this, but a number that don't support it. (Posner, 1977, in the Course Reader)

From the evidence of the rest of this article, no other doctor was quite so forthright about the fact that some aspects of medical treatment are founded as much on faith as knowledge. They hinted at this, but they did not openly state it. In this sort of study the researcher is a kind of detective who has to rely on fragments, hints and half-concealed clues. Armed with the insight provided by this one doctor, the researcher interprets what others have to say in a new light. Posner underlines the key phrases so that the reader may do the same. This is obviously a difficult mode of inquiry and can sometimes lead to gross misinterpretation. However, as we have seen, all interview studies face problems. To rely simply on the frequency with which things are said is often to be naïve. Posner shows how alternative methods can be most revealing.

One other feature of the extract does however deserve some comment. Posner uses this quotation to show that there are 'magical' elements to the practice of modern medicine. But if you examine the doctor's statement closely, there are other things he says that are wholly characteristic of science and not like magic at all.

☐ Which phrases strike you as typical of a scientific approach?
■ The key phrases are 'evidence', 'not weighted heavily in favour', 'if ... should', 'no outstanding evidence', 'true', 'a number of papers that support this, but a number that don't'. These illustrate the scientific themes of complexity, doubt, weighing evidence carefully, and the search for truth.

So, just as it can pay to check the tables in papers with numerical data, it is always worth giving the quotations in qualitative papers a second glance. Do they fully support the author's argument or are there unanalysed features that point in different directions? Readers as well as researchers can be detectives.

Focusing down

Given the problems of determining what people do from what they say, interviews present several problems of interpretation. Some qualitative researchers prefer to focus on the systematic recording of action rather than on reports of action. For example, consultations between doctors and patients can be recorded in detail by verbatim notes, by audiotape and by videotape. Paper and pencil leaves out a lot but enables a large number of occasions to be analysed. Videotape provides the most detail; so much so that only a small number of cases can be handled. Once the data have been gathered, the researcher looks for *patterns*.

Here, as examples, are two extracts from paediatric consultations, one from the United States, the other from Scotland. Consider the similarities and differences between them. (That with doctor A is, by the way, very far from typical.)

Extract 1

DOCTOR A   What do you wash her diapers [nappies] in?
MOTHER   Ivory Snow.
DOCTOR A   Why do you use Ivory Snow?
MOTHER   Well, its supposed to make the diapers softer than other washing powders.
DOCTOR A   How do you know Ivory Snow makes diapers softer?
MOTHER   [*shrugs awkwardly*] Well, um ... [*mumbles something about her mother and advertisements*].
DOCTOR A   You don't want to believe everything you see in the adverts. It's a business. That's *their* business; *your* business is your baby. [*She then explains that the rash is due to ammonia in the urine and that Ivory Snow is too weak. The mother should use an ordinary washing powder.*]
MOTHER   I do put vinegar in it.
DOCTOR A   [*amazed*] Why do you do that?
MOTHER   Well I was told.
DOCTOR A   Who told you?
MOTHER   My mother did.
DOCTOR A   What difference does it make?
MOTHER   Well, she said ... I thought it ...
DOCTOR A   It doesn't do any good at all. (Strong, 1979, p.43)

Extract 2

DOCTOR B   And you feed him [6-month old baby] on Farex?
MOTHER   In the morning and evening.
DOCTOR B   And porridge.
MOTHER   Aye.
DOCTOR B   Does he get anything else for elevenses?
MOTHER   Just biscuits.
DOCTOR B   How much porridge does he get?
MOTHER   Oh, nae much.
DOCTOR B   How much does he get at lunch-time?
MOTHER   Oh, just mince and tatties.
DOCTOR B   Do you give him anything mid-afternoon?
MOTHER   No.

DOCTOR B   And what does he get for his tea?

MOTHER   Oh, a boiled egg or a scrambled egg.

DOCTOR B   And this is as well as milk?

MOTHER   Aye [*rest inaudible*].

DOCTOR B   Well, I think he's putting on a bit too much weight. Is he fatter than your other children?

MOTHER   Aye.

DOCTOR B   If I were you, I'd miss out the Farex and the porridge at breakfast and the biscuit as well. It's best to do this now because if children get fat now then they tend to be fatter later on in life. He's supposed to be twice his birthweight now and he's a good bit more than that, isn't he? This is very important. He's putting on a bit too much weight. (Strong, 1979, pp.46 and 47)

Both extracts follow a question/answer sequence in which, with only one exception, the doctor asks all the questions, and only the doctor comments on what the mother has said. Both consultations involve delicate matters: the children's problems might be seen as partly the mother's responsibility. There are, however, important differences. Doctor A's consultation is a cross-examination. She wants to know *why* the mother has done things. Doctor B merely asks *what* the mother has done. To search for motives when a person's 'guilt' has already been established, must be done with delicacy if they are not to be further discredited. To ask about actions as opposed to reasons is much less threatening.

□   How accurately do these quotations represent the real flavour of interaction?

■   Real interaction is a matter of posture, gesture and eye-contact as well as speech. Accent, pitch and tone are also important. Also, the quotations omit the 'ums' and 'ers'; the speakers do not overlap; everything seems to make sense. These features are characteristic of written speech, and not of spoken language.

These transcripts were based on notes; those about doctor B were taken at the time; those with doctor A constructed immediately afterwards. But even with tape-recording, there are problems with transcription. The more one listens to speech, the more complex it becomes. The quotations in most research reports are highly simplified. The subtleties of speech are turned into the kind of smooth prose that novelists write but that we never hear or speak. (Test this out for yourself by trying to transcribe two or three minutes of recorded talk.)

This brief survey of qualitative methods has had to omit several important sources of qualitative data. We have barely touched on the array of written sources of information. There are also pictures or images. Finally, there are other sorts of material objects or remains. (Hospital architecture, for example, is a rewarding field of study.)

Let us focus on the most important of these, *written sources*. Most events occur without the benefit of an observing social scientist. However, an enormous number of transactions do require some form of written record. There are also some things that exist only in and through writing — teaching like this and medical journals, for example. There is, therefore, a mountain of data in libraries and archives. These data may be categorised more formally into: (a) personal documents — diaries and letters; (b) published commentary, reporting and analysis; and (c) official documents — medical records, parish registers, the minutes of health authority meetings, memoranda, official letters and government reports.

□   Written materials present the same problem of interpretation as do observational and interview methods. What are these problems?

■   Personal or official records are shaped by the interests of the writer and the audience, just as social science observations and interviews are.

□   What kind of people and actions are most likely to be recorded in this fashion?

■   In general, it is the powerful, the literate, the official and the deviant whose lives are most likely to be recorded by themselves or by others. Historical documents are therefore biased towards the actions and concerns of the elite. How to study everyone else — 'history from below' — is a problem that has increasingly engaged researchers over the past fifty years. Interviewing the elderly — *oral history* — is a popular solution for the recent past.

Objective for Chapter 9

When you have studied this chapter, you should be able to:

9.1 Describe some of the principal forms of qualitative research and compare their various uses, advantages and disadvantages.

Question for Chapter 9

1 (*Objective 9.1*) The following interaction was recorded in a hospital clinic.

> A paediatrician is speaking to a mother wanting to adopt a baby and to the social worker who has accompanied her. He has just carried out the necessary examination of the baby and completed the adoption form for the magistrate. 'I certainly think everything's all right ... I can't find any abnormalities so it'll be through by the end of January....' After they have left, he comments to the researcher, 'That was a difficult one. I'd have been a lot happier if she'd reacted to the rattle and lifted her head up earlier. She did it in the end but I felt she could have done it earlier. One has also got to take into account that she is an Indian baby; they might be slower to develop. Negroes, of course, are faster. There's also the reason why she's adopting this baby. She may be one of those people who have a thing about under-privileged children. I would like to see her again in two or three months' time perhaps, but as she seems to be so set on this thing, I won't implant the doubt in her mind. She seemed a pretty lively thing.'
> (Strong, 1979, pp.174 and 175)

Now answer the following questions:

(a) Does this seem like real speech? Is it likely to have been accurately transcribed?

(b) Would you classify the doctor's second speech as observational or interview data?

(c) We noted earlier, that people do not necessarily alter their behaviour if an observer is present. Is this true here?

(d) As we saw earlier, both qualitative research and lay speech contain all kinds of primitive forms of quantification. What quantitative statements can you detect in what the doctor has to say? (Look hard.)

(e) What does this quote tell us about the trustworthiness of official records, such as adoption forms?

10
Quantitative social research

Qualitative methods can tell us many things about the social world. They also have many drawbacks. Social scientists should quantify wherever this is possible. Some key techniques for doing this were discussed in Chapters 4–6 (statistics and epidemiology). Some other methods, such as the costing and mathematical modelling used by economists, are too technical to be considered here. But something else is still needed. Observation and interview can be conducted by numerical as well as qualitative means. Which should we choose? And when? Also, we have emphasised the special difficulties of measuring the social world. How can we overcome these? This needs thought.

Observational studies

A good example of the numerical approach to the observation of behaviour is a study conducted in the 1960s by an American sociologist, Murray Melbin (1969). His particular interest was the bizarre behaviour of some mental patients. When did it happen and why? To study this, Melbin first defined precisely what he meant by 'bizarre', and then trained observers in this definition. They watched for two-hour periods in different areas of two mental hospitals — one a small private institution, the other a much larger public hospital. The latter had fifteen times as many patients, but relatively fewer psychiatrists; perhaps to compensate for this it used more drug therapy. The siting and timing of the observation were carefully randomised. Observation lasted 48 hours in the private hospital, 56 hours in the State hospital. The results are given in Table 10.1.

Table 10.1 Bizarre episodes recorded in two mental hospitals

	Time of episode	
	weekdays	evenings/weekend
private hospital	34	17
State hospital	27	19

(data from Melbin, 1969, p.653)

☐ Relatively speaking, when and where did bizarre episodes occur most frequently?

■ The private hospital experienced bizarre episodes much more frequently than the State hospital. (Remember there were fifteen times more patients in the State hospital.) In both institutions, such episodes were more common on weekdays than in the evenings or at weekends.

☐ What might explain these differences? (Think back over what you know about the drug therapy and the psychiatrists.)

■ There are three plausible explanations. One is not mentioned by Melbin. The different hospitals might have very different sorts of patient. We are not told; though even if they do, this does not explain the variation in the timing of the episodes. However, the difference might also be to do with the variation in drug therapy. We know that the two hospitals differed in this, and perhaps patients were given more drugs in the evenings and at weekends. Melbin himself suggests a third, intriguing possibility: that the association is with the presence of psychiatrists. There were far more psychiatrists on duty during weekdays than at other times, and the private hospital had a far higher staff–patient ratio. Viewed in this light, episodes of bizarre behaviour may possibly be a plea for help by the desperate.

As you saw from the discussion of the clinical method, changes in the frequency of relatively common events are hard to spot. (Remember the example of the parrots and sparrows.) Bizarre behaviour is not unusual in mental hospitals, so it may need careful quantification to spot changes in its incidence.

Interview studies

Numerical observation studies are comparatively rare in social science; most are found in psychology. But the numerical form of the interview, the *survey, questionnaire* or *structured interview* is found in every walk of modern life. Postal questionnaires are cheap but can ask only a limited number of questions. Face-to-face interviews are more expensive but produce more data. Telephone interviews, an increasingly popular method, come somewhere in between. However conducted, such surveys have two main characteristics: the questions and many of the answers are fixed in advance and everyone is asked the same question and must normally choose their answer from a given set of alternatives. (A modified form, called 'semi-structured', comes half-way between this and the informal interview.)

☐ What are the advantages of the survey method compared with informal interviewing?
■ Because the questions and answers are fixed, one can interview very large numbers of people in a uniform fashion and count the answers with ease. It is therefore possible to get systematic information from an adequate sample of the population in question. Data from informal interviews are often too diffuse for easy quantification and taken from too small a number of people to be fully representative.

The survey method also has some disadvantages. The questions are fixed and the interviewees cannot normally answer in their own words; both can result in distortion. Surveys should be limited to relatively simple questions. Informal methods cope better with detail and complexity.

These points can be taken further. The following quotations are from a questionnaire study by Ann Cartwright and Anne Bowling, two British sociologists. (A further extract from their work can be found in the Course Reader, Part 6, Section 6.5.)

The widowed were asked what they felt about the care and treatment their spouse had from their general practitioner before their death and then to sum up whether this care was 'very good', 'fairly good', or 'not very good' ... 8 per cent had no contact with a general practitioner in the year before their death. For the others, in two thirds, the care was felt to be 'very good', a quarter of the widowed described it as 'fairly good' and a tenth as 'not very good'. (Cartwright and Bowling, 1982, p.25)

Just over half (53%) of the deaths in our sample took place in hospital. In addition, 44 per cent of those dying at home were admitted to hospital at some time during the last quarter of their lives, so altogether three-quarters, 74 per cent of these married people, spent some part of their last year in hospital. But few were there for long. Only a small minority, 8 per cent had spent three months or longer in hospital. (Cartwright and Bowling, 1982, pp.19 and 20)

☐ The types of information discussed in these two quotations present distinctly different problems of interpretation. What are these?
■ The meaning of 'good' can vary enormously. Those who gave apparently similar answers might have meant very different things by them. And what we find 'fairly good' now, we might find 'excellent' later, or vice versa. By contrast, the information asked for in the second question is clearly knowable and capable of precise definition. (Whether people actually know it is another question.)

Attempting to poll satisfaction is still a useful exercise. Nevertheless, fixing the precise shape of questions and answers in advance can create problems. Are the questions sufficiently precise? Is the set of possible responses reasonable? Or, are there silly answers to silly questions?

Two other matters also need checking. How were people chosen for interviewing? Was care taken to ensure that they were representative of the wider groups under study? Some of the benefits of random sampling were discussed earlier when studies of spina bifida were considered. The same lessons apply here. But not all surveys follow these rules. One of the most famous questionnaire studies was conducted in the 1950s by Alfred Kinsey (another entomologist!) and his colleagues on the sexual practices of American adults (Kinsey *et al.*, 1948 and 1953). The sample was obtained by advertising for volunteers in a local newspaper.

☐ How might advertising for subjects have affected the 'Kinsey Report'?
■ It seems unlikely that those who volunteered to be interviewed about their sexual habits were representative of the general public.

Kinsey compounded the error by calling his studies, *Sexual Behavior in the Human Male* and *Sexual Behavior in the Human Female*.

☐ Why are these titles misleading?
■ Americans are not a representative sample of the human race.

The third thing to check is the response rate, the proportion of people who replied to the questionnaire.

☐ What is the importance of checking the response rate?
■ Willingness or ability to reply is not random, but often influenced by class, age, and so on. Even if the initial sample were randomly selected, a low response rate may bias the results.

Devising measures

When William the Conqueror had finished conquering, he ordered a detailed survey of all the property in his new kingdom — the 'Domesday Book'. How much, precisely, had he got? As this example shows, measuring the social world is done for administrative and political reasons as well as a disinterested love of knowledge. The figures produced are conventionally known as 'statistics'. (The other, more technical, meaning of statistics refers to a branch of mathematics, not to the numbers themselves.) 'Statistics' are cited everywhere in modern life, and every organisation studies itself, its clientele and its environment through numerical means. Developing accurate measures is therefore of great social, economic and political importance. For precisely the same reasons, there is a powerful, sometimes dubious, incentive for bureaucracies to prefer some measures to others.

☐ Try to list some aspects of the social world whose definition and measurement are currently controversial.
■ Social class, health, profits, intelligence, ethnicity, the money supply and mental illness are all examples. You may have thought of others.

Unlike liquid in a measuring jug, none of these things can be measured directly. We need instead to find *'proxy'* (or indirect) *measures*. The process of developing such measures has the hideous name of *operationalisation*. But besides its name, operationalisation has several more important problems, which we shall illustrate through the example of social class.

☐ You may recall our earlier discussion of Mr Lawson's social class. How did it affect his diabetes?
■ Reference was made to income, diet and smoking. You might have added education, conditions at work, drinking habits, ownership of a car or telephone, family size and wealth, plus more abstract concepts such as power and status.

So 'social class' refers to a number of separate things. In Marxist theory a person's class is defined by whether or not they own 'capital', that is, the resources for economic production such as a factory. Other theories use much broader definitions, covering many of the topics noted above. There is in fact an enormous literature on the meaning of social class, a literature so complex and controversial that it presents the quantitative researcher with a difficult problem. If we want to measure class we have to choose a precise definition — but which one?

Operationalisation usually means making the best of a bad job. As such, researchers are strongly influenced by what has been done in previous studies. If the proxy for x has traditionally been y, then whatever the problems with

y, there are powerful reasons for choosing it yet again. At least the results will be compatible with those of previous research. In the area of social class this has led to distinct national traditions. In Britain social class is normally defined using occupation as the major proxy measure. The British tradition was begun in 1911 by the government department in charge of the census. Its officials wanted to estimate the social class of every person in the country, so the measure had to be quick, easy and reliable. A *reliable* definition (a technical term) is one on which almost everyone agrees. It can therefore be used in the same way by different people at different times — exactly what is needed for a huge operation like the census. Occupation fits the bill. Most occupations have special names and are easy to distinguish, and because of this occupation is used by the great majority of British academic researchers and government agencies.

☐ Can one now go ahead and use occupation to measure social class?
■ No.
☐ Why not? What does one need to know first?
■ Occupation may be easy to measure, but is it a measure of social class? In technical terms, measures need to be *valid* as well as reliable.

As there is no agreement about what social class is, there can never be a truly valid measure of it. We must settle for second-best. However, there are several reasons for thinking that an occupational measure does get at some important aspects of social class.

Let us begin by examining the modern version of the scheme used by the census. This scheme, called the 'Registrar General's Social Classes' allocates people to five categories or social classes, class III being further divided into manual and non-manual workers. The groups included in each were selected to ensure that:

so far as is possible, each category is homogeneous in relation to the basic criterion of the general standing within the community of the occupations concerned. This criterion is naturally correlated with, and its application conditioned by, other factors such as education and economic environment, but it has no direct relationship to the average level of remuneration of particular occupations. Each occupational unit group has been assigned as a whole to a Social Class, and is not a specific assignment of individuals based on the merits of a particular case.

The Social Class appropriate to any combination of occupation and status is derived by the following rules:
(a) each occupation is given a basic Social Class

[see Table 10.2 for some examples]

(b) persons of foreman status whose basic Social Class is IV or V are allotted to Social Class III

(c) persons of manager status are allocated either to Social Class II or III, the latter applying if the basic class is IV or V. (The Registrar General, 1970)

□ What criterion is given for this particular ranking of occupations?

■ The criterion is 'the general standing within the community of the occupations concerned'. The definition of social class is therefore based on an analysis of *status*.

Status is only one of the many aspects of the meaning of social class and, according to some theories, not an important one. But the man who first developed this classification in 1921, T.H.C. Stevenson, did something else as well. The association between occupation and life-expectancy had long been known. Stevenson showed that his six social classes, ranked on the basis of occupational prestige, were also associated with different mortality rates, rising from a low rate in class I to a high one in class V.

Given its links with both status and mortality, occupation seems to be quite a useful measure of social class, though the general concept includes a good many other matters. However, think a little more about particular occupations. Consider a list of some of the main dimensions of social class that are measured, at least in part, by occupation.

1 Share of economic production.
2 Personal control over time and activities.
3 Mortality.
4 Intellectual and personal development.
5 Security of tenure in employment.
6 Prestige.

□ What are some of the ways members of different occupations do more or less well in terms of this list? (Think for example, of the way in which a university lecturer and a hospital cleaner would differ.)

■ Different occupations would differ in some of the following ways: (i) share of economic production — income, ownership of property and other durables, fringe benefits; (ii) personal control over time and activities — decision-making, rights to take a holiday or other leave, rights to allocate free time, and to choose where to work and when; (iii) mortality — health and safety at work; (iv) intellectual and personal development — education and training opportunities, scope for individual fulfilment, pleasure and enjoyment; (v) security of tenure in employment — risk of unemployment, starting date, full-time or part-time, etc; (vi) prestige — amount of social status attaching to occupation.

So *occupation* refers to power and opportunity as well as to status and mortality. There are, however, yet more problems with the use of occupation as a measure of social class.

Table 10.2 Typical occupations* by social class

Social class	Examples of occupations included*
I Professional, etc.	accountant, architect, chemist, company secretary, doctor, engineer, judge, lawyer, optician, scientist, solicitor, surveyor, university teacher
II Intermediate	aircraft pilot or engineer, chiropodist, farmer, laboratory assistant or technician, manager, proprietor, publican, member of parliament, nurse, pilot or fire-brigade officer, schoolteacher
III (N.) Skilled non-manual	auctioneer, cashier, clerical worker, commercial traveller, draughtsman, estate agent, sales representative, secretary, shop assistant, typist, telephone supervisor
III (M.) Skilled manual	baker, bus driver, butcher, bricklayer, carpenter, cook, electrician, hairdresser, miner (underground), policeman or fireman, railway engine driver/guard, upholsterer
IV Partly skilled	agricultural worker, barman, bus conductor, fisherman, hospital orderly, machine sewer, packer, postman, roundsman, street vendor, telephone operator
V Unskilled	charwoman, chimney sweep, kitchen hand, labourer, lorry driver's mate, office cleaner, railway porter, van guards, window cleaner

*In alphabetical order. These are mainly basic occupation titles; foremen and managers in many occupations listed are allotted to different classes. (The Registrar General, 1970)

□ Re-examine the Registrar General's scheme and list some other problems associated with it.

■ Some of the job titles look rather old-fashioned. Some of the rankings look most odd — do you know an estate agent who would be happy to be classed as III non-manual, for example? And what happens to people who do not have paid occupations: housewives, the elderly, children, prisoners and the chronically sick? And if one wants to assign families and households to social classes, whose occupation should be used? Finally, the Registrar General ranks occupation on the basis of what has been described as the 'pecking order traditionally associated with men's jobs'.

Let us take just one of these issues, that of gender. Many argue that the current convention of classifying households on the basis of the man's occupation is inadequate. The classification also ignores the major differences between men and women in the kinds of paid employment they get. Look at Table 10.3.

Table 10.3 Percentages of married women and 'single' women in each social class, as measured by their own and their husband's occupations

| Social class | Married | | Single, widowed and divorced |
	own occupation	husband's occupation	
I	0.9	5.3	1.2
II	16.2	19.8	19.2
III skilled non-manual	35.4	11.3	41.2
III skilled manual	10.0	39.0	10.8
IV	28.2	17.5	22.7
V	9.4	7.1	4.9

(*Social Trends*, 1975, p.6)

□ Where do women's jobs cluster in Table 10.3? What does this indicate?

■ Women's jobs are concentrated into social classes III skilled non-manual and IV — possibly because these are the only jobs women can get. But some people argue that the Registrar General's ranking does not discriminate well between women's jobs.

Finally, what about the huge number of women whose work consists of unpaid domestic labour? Such work is an important contribution to our standard of living, but those who do it, because they are unpaid, are still officially classed as 'economically inactive'.

It is, however, possible to defend the Registrar General's position on the classification of women. Some people acknowledge that the scheme does treat women as mere

appendages of men, but argue that this is in fact the way our society treats women. The fault lies not in the classification but in the reality that it measures. The second argument concerns the kind of evidence Stevenson used to validate his original scheme, evidence of mortality. A recent study of a sample of people from the 1971 Census suggests that if class is measured by the wives' occupation then women in social classes IV and V had a slightly lower mortality rate than those in classes I and II. This may possibly be true, but it certainly seems odd. However, when they looked at married women in a particular class — III skilled non-manual — and then examined the relationship of their mortality rate to their husband's occupation a different picture emerged (Table 10.4).

Table 10.4 The mortality (SMR) of two groups of married women aged 15–74 as ranked by their husband's social class

| Husband's social class | Married women | |
	employed, social class III skilled non-manual	housewives (inactive)
I	72	55
II	88	89
III skilled non-manual	94	79
III skilled manual	98	101
IV	119	102
V	117	130
(Armed Forces, inadequately described and unoccupied)	—	138

(Fox and Goldblatt, 1982, Table 3.12. The reference populations used for standardising the mortality of the two groups of women were, respectively, *all* class III non-manual women and *all* 'inactive' women in the sample studied.)

□ What is the relationship of their husband's social class to the women's mortality in Table 10.4?

■ This is the normal pattern, with mortality lowest in class I and highest in class V.

□ What does this suggest?

■ It suggests that whatever the relationship between the women's occupations and their mortality, if they are married, their husbands' social class exerts a powerful effect.

Such evidence does not settle the debate. It is clear that the present occupational method of measuring class is designed for men and not women. As a compromise, many researchers now classify married women by both their own and their husband's occupations and check what difference this makes.

One final note: there is no need to use just one measure when trying to operationalise a concept. Melbin used several criteria for bizarre behaviour, and it is possible to do the same for social class. In the United States, income and education are commonly combined. In Britain, a few researchers have tried adding to occupation, education, type of housing, area of residence, and so on. These add refinement. They are also more costly, whereas occupational data are easy to collect and simple to handle. Moreover, this increasing sophistication does not fundamentally alter the final outcome.

Objectives for Chapter 10

Now that you have studied this chapter, you should be able to:

10.1 Discuss the advantages and disadvantages of quantitative social research and of structured interviews in particular.

10.2 Identify some of the difficulties associated with developing proxy measures for — or operationalising — aspects of the social world.

Questions for Chapter 10

1 *(Objective 10.1)* A local authority social services department is planning to develop a home-help service. They want to assess how many of the elderly people living alone in the borough might need such support and what type of support they need most. They decide to use a questionnaire.

(a) What might be their reasons for using a questionnaire?

(b) What would be the best way to deliver the questionnaire to the old people: (i) face to face, (ii) through the post, or (iii) by telephone?

2 *(Objective 10.2)* A group of researchers have decided to try to measure how independent the old people they are interviewing are. Comment on some of the difficulties they may face as they try to measure — or operationalise — independence and what factors they need to consider.

11
Science: facts, theories and values

In this chapter, we want to introduce you to some of the problems of building theories and models to 'fit' the evidence we collect. We shall then look more carefully at a particular issue that has run right through this book, but until now we have side-stepped: the problem of what we mean by the word 'cause', and what might be the relationship between biological and social definitions of 'cause'. Finally, we consider the complexities of the relationship between biological and social explanations in terms of one, much misunderstood, concept, that of race.

About hypotheses

Let us begin with the problem of making scientific hypotheses. Medicine, as you have seen, sets problems that scientists try to answer (such as what causes diabetes?).

☐ List some of the organising assumptions used by Banting and Best in making their experiments and forming hypotheses about the role of the pancreas in diabetes (from Chapters 2 and 3).

■ There are a large number, but your list should include at least some of the following:

1 There is a disease state, a single entity called 'diabetes mellitus'.

2 The correct way to study diabetes is to seek inside the bodies of the sufferers themselves rather than to look for factors in the environment or diet that might be responsible.

3 Animals such as dogs can form 'model systems' in which to study human disease.

4 If pancreatic juice alleviated the symptoms of diabetes then this must be because it contained a particular active substance that could be purified — the hormone insulin.

5 If insulin alleviated the symptoms of diabetes, this was because the disease was caused by lack of insulin.

This reductionist scientific method is committed to concepts of individual diseases. Hence, medicine seeks to define disease-entities as collections of signs and symptoms, and biology then locates the 'causes' of these entities in specific phenomena, such as genetic abnormality, infectious microorganisms, or whatever.

Yet time and time again one comes across what seem to be conflicting or mutually exclusive interpretations of the causes of the phenomena of health and disease. How is one to distinguish between or reconcile such apparently conflicting theories or explanations for diseases, from the common cold to schizophrenia?

About causes

Let us begin with reductionism, the belief that we can understand, explain and predict the behaviour of complex systems, such as humans, in terms of their component parts. Reductionism is both a *method* — a way of doing experiments, as in the examples in Chapter 3 — and a *philosophy*, a belief that the ultimate explanation of a phenomenon is given by analysis of its components. Methodologically, reductionism has proved an immensely powerful tool; but it is now time to consider its philosophical limitations.

Consider some of the ways in which we have used the word 'cause' in previous chapters. For instance:

☐ What did we suggest was the cause of diabetes, scurvy and pellagra in Chapter 3?

■ The causes suggested were: insulin deficiency (diabetes), vitamin C deficiency (scurvy) and vitamin B deficiency (pellagra).

Now think back to the example of scurvy and let us ask the same question in a broader framework.

☐ Why did the sailors on Captain Cook's ship become affected with scurvy? (Think about why the sailors were there.)

■ Yes, lack of vitamin C is part of the answer. But if the sailors had not been press-ganged into service on a long sea voyage, they would not have found themselves in a situation in which they were likely to suffer a deficiency of vitamin C.

And that long sea voyage was an aspect of Britain's economic, social and political expansion during the eighteenth century, the search for colonies and markets abroad that led the British Admiralty to commission Captain Cook's voyage. And the dietary conditions on the ships were part of a system of class relations that saw the sailors only as 'hands' to perform particular tasks on board. Are these not equally to be taken into account as the causes of the sailor's scurvy?

☐ Now, what *causes* pellagra? (Apply the same approach in answering.)

■ Pellagra is caused by a lack of vitamin B in the diet of the poor in the southern states of the USA, of course. But what caused that lack, when, as we have said, the mill-hands but not the mill-owners were those who were affected? Clearly, the inadequate diet is itself one aspect of a division in society between rich and poor; again the causes of pellagra are not 'only' biological. The 'cure' for pellagra could be to feed those suffering from it special supplements of vitamin B pills — or it could be to pay them higher wages so that they could afford the food the mill-owners took for granted.

☐ Can you now apply the same logic to the *cause* of diabetes?

■ This answer might seem less obvious. Mr Lawson's lack of insulin, which produced the symptoms labelled diabetes, did not seem to be, on the basis of the information we gave you, the result of social circumstances. It seemed to arise from internal factors in his biological makeup, perhaps his genes. But we have noted that many people with sugar in their urine who show up as 'positive' on biochemical tests, do not show other clinical signs of the disease. Also, not everyone with low insulin suffers the disease; much depends on diet. So we must question why Mr Lawson developed diabetes when others with sugar in their urine did not.

There is evidence that diabetes is on the increase in the UK today. There is an association between the amount of diabetes in the population and measures of wealth such as gross national product. Perhaps the increase is linked to dietary changes such as the increased amount of sugar as opposed to starch in our daily food intake. This change in its turn is related to complex structures of farming

subsidies, the policies of the great multinational food companies, and so forth. Treating Mr Lawson's diabetes with insulin injections is a way of helping him overcome his problem, and therefore part of the doctor's responsibility. But reducing the prevalence of diabetes in the population as a whole, like reducing pellagra, requires a much broader approach. Apart from anything else, treating diabetes successfully increases its *incidence* in the population, both because the affected people live longer, and also because diabetes tends to be inherited. This means more diabetics live long enough to have children who themselves have a good chance of being affected.

You can now begin to see some of the complexities embedded in the concepts of *cause* and of *treatment* for diseases. Any individual can be viewed as being at the meeting point of biological, or internal causes, and of social or external causes. This relationship can be illustrated as in Figure 11.1. In the diagram, we have introduced a new

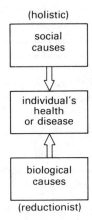

Figure 11.1

phrase to describe the 'top-down' type of social explanation: we refer to it as '*holistic*', to contrast it with the reductionism of the 'bottom-up' type of explanation. Holistic explanations describe the individual's health or disease as a product of the social system in which they are embedded. (Note that the term 'holistic' is popularly used in a number of different ways, all antithetical to reductionism but carrying a variety of extra meanings; here, we mean only to contrast 'top-down' and 'bottom-up' types of explanation of the phenomena of health and disease.)

But are top-down/bottom-up explanations sufficient? Instead of talking about 'any individual' as a product of biological and social causes, ask yourself, 'Can I regard *myself* as a product of social and biological causes alone?' Most people would find such a description inadequate. They would want to include in a description of themselves a sense of their own personal history and personal identity.

If people feel sick — 'not themselves' — it is a feeling experienced with the whole body and consciousness simultaneously.

☐ Supposing you were to slip at work and break a leg, and feel acute pain as a result. What would be the cause of the pain of the broken leg?

■ In biological terms, the pain is caused by a blow to a particular bone, its fracture and the consequent activation of nerves responsible for sensing pain. But how did the leg come to be broken? Those offering social causes might talk about the conditions under which you were working: maybe a worn carpet, too little light or too little room between machines.

But you would also think to yourself: 'If only I wasn't so absent-minded and had been looking where I was going.' 'If only I hadn't been angry or upset.' 'If only I hadn't had so much to drink the night before.' By thinking in this way, you are explaining your broken leg in terms of things you were feeling at the time or things that had occurred in your past. That is, you are seeking for a cause in your own personal history, within which is included both what has happened in your life and also your own personal psychological makeup, your own consciousness of who you are as a person and how you have come to be like this. Personal life history is thus another major dimension to the explanation of, and the search for, the causes of health and disease. Let us amend Figure 11.1 therefore, to look like Figure 11.2.

Because personal explanations relate to an individual's past, they bring the dimension of time into explanations of health and disease — whether the immediate past of yesterday's hangover or the remote past of childhood or developmental experience. They are temporal causes. Although all causes speak of the present and the past, everyone is concerned with the fact that they are moving steadily into the future: medicine is therefore concerned

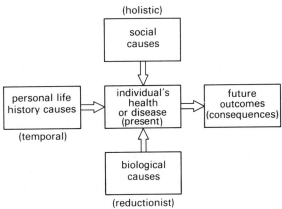

Figure 11.3

with prospects and with outcomes. So, for symmetry, we can complete the diagram as in Figure 11.3.

One of the main goals of this course is to bring about an understanding of how these different types of cause can be integrated and what relationship they have to future outcomes. But can they be integrated? It is readily understood that they must all interact in some complex manner that can be partly predicted, and that it is not possible to obtain a complete picture of an individual's present state or future trajectory without taking this interaction into account. But also each type of cause has found its own special domain of study, its own way of looking at the world and the place of human beings within it.

It is often not easy to see the relationship between biological and social explanations, and harder still to see how they relate to those offered by psychology, which is the study of personal history. Partly because of the way in which these disciplines have grown up separately, each with their own set of blinkers, there are problems in relating them. But science in general is also committed to the thesis of the unity of knowledge: in the material world social causes are simultaneously biological and personal; personal causes are simultaneously biological and social; biological causes are simultaneously personal and social; even though the ways in which these links may be drawn can be very difficult to see in practice.

Facts and theories

Now let us explore another issue in the methodology of both natural and social sciences, which may not be as obvious as it might seem at first sight: the relationships between 'facts' and 'theories'. To begin to see what the problem is, consider again that consultation between the doctor and Mr Lawson with which we began Chapter 2.

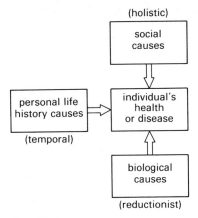

Figure 11.2

What do we know of it? The doctor could give one account and Mr Lawson another. Their accounts would agree in places but be subtly different in others. Whom are we to believe? Biology and scientific medicine tend to favour the objective statement of the doctor. The qualitative methods of social science have more space for subjectivity. One could consult the doctor's case notes, a primary 'objective' source. But by the time the doctor came to write up Mr Lawson's case for a research paper, her viewpoint would again have shifted: certain features would be emphasised at the expense of others, depending on the point the doctor was trying to make. If the doctor became famous as a result of the case and wrote her autobiography 30 years later, her recollection would again have subtly modified the account. And by the time the case appeared in medical textbooks, it would have changed once more. If ideas about the causes of diabetes were later reconsidered by scientists who had other theories, or in the light of new evidence, the case notes would be re-evaluated from yet another perspective. Thus, the very facts seem elusive and under dispute even before they become refracted by theory.

As you read through Chapters 3–10 you will have become aware of the many different ways in which 'facts' can be collected and expressed. Indeed, there is a sense in which facts do not exist in the absence of a theory within which they are framed. Even facts about the numbers of people born or dying each year take shape from the way in which they are expressed.

If the very 'facts' are elusive, what about the theories within which facts are assembled, discussed and explained? Theories are attempts to generalise, to make rules about how to describe the world and to give people some capacity to predict the outcomes of events. Theories are often metaphors, ways of explaining part of the world as if it were like some other part. Nineteenth-century physicists studied atoms 'as if' they were billiard balls, twentieth-century neuroscientists study brains 'as if' they were mainframe computers. Banting and Best studied diabetic dogs 'as if' they were humans.

Scientific theories change and transmute; at best scientific 'truth' is only historically relative, even without new 'facts' becoming available. It is clear from all accounts of 'scientific progress' that newly discovered facts can change theories profoundly. Before 1953, biologists were convinced that the most important molecules present in living organisms were proteins, and that because of this it would turn out that genes, the units of heredity, were protein. A number of key experiments had suggested that the genetic material might not be protein at all but quite another substance, the nucleic acid DNA. But DNA was believed to be rather an inert, uninteresting molecule, until in 1953 Crick and Watson published a paper revealing that the structure of DNA was eminently suited to a process of self-replication (Watson and Crick, 1953).* This made it an immediate candidate to be 'the' genetic material. At once the old experiments were reinterpreted, and within a few years DNA theory had become the conventional wisdom of the new molecular biology. The new theory 'drove' new experiments: questions became interesting that were boring or meaningless before, in the old 'protein' days, and many questions that had previously seemed of central importance ceased to be of interest.

But where do the new theories come from? They are based on metaphors and inevitably scientists devise these metaphors out of their own experience. Again, an example from the history of biology will show how this works. All cells use energy, derived from burning sugar (glucose). Burning this sugar, it was shown during the 1930s, generates a substance, called ATP for short, which is in turn used up in the complex reactions by which the cell either synthesises new molecules (proteins for instance) or performs work on the world as a muscle or gland. Analysing cell energetics and energy flow became the key task of biochemistry in the 1930s and 1940s, and the discoverer of ATP used the explicit metaphor of ATP as the cell's 'energy currency'. On strict 'monetarist' principles, the cell could only 'spend' the ATP it 'earned' by burning glucose. This 'economic model' of the cell was replaced in the 1950s with a new set of metaphors focused not around the exchange of *energy*, but around the exchange of *information*. Interest shifted to the study of DNA, the genetic material that was seen as an 'information molecule' carrying instructions across the generations. Cell processes were no longer analysed in terms of the 1930s power station or factory, but according to models of management, feedback, control processes and information transfer, which were more appropriate to the sophisticated modern world. The biologists had explicitly borrowed models derived from economics and social theories to describe the properties of cells and to organise subsequent experiments.

☐   What are some other metaphors used in biology and medicine to describe the functions of the human body?
■   A few of them are the heart as a pump, the brain as a computer, the kidneys and bladder as water-works and the immune system as a task force.

Science, therefore, does not proceed in a social vacuum. Despite the claim of some scientists and philosophers, even natural science is not 'neutral' in its account of the world. Scientists are driven to answer questions 'set' by social need

* You will understand this more fully, if you know no biology, when you come to study, *The Biology of Health and Disease*. (U205, Book IV)

— for instance, the 'cause' of disease — along paths constrained by theories that are themselves derived from the experience of the social world in which scientists live and work. And yet science claims to be a truthful description of the real material world. That is its paradox, and its power. For in the last analysis science is a method of describing and acting upon the real material world, and its list of 'facts' and its changing theories have to be matched against that real world. If the theories cannot describe it, if the 'facts' turn out to be misrepresentations or only partial descriptions, then they have a short life only. Yet if the cell is described in terms of 'energy currency' and in terms of 'information flow' which is the description that better matches the real world — or are both only partial metaphors, reflections seen in a distorting mirror of social expectations? Perhaps both ways of interpreting the cell are equally 'true' and which is judged the better choice depends only on the answers one expects. If you want to know about the mechanisms of heredity, energy flow is not important; if you want to know why you get cramp and become breathless if you run hard, then information flow is irrelevant.

The nature of science

At this stage it is important to reconsider just what is contained in that word we have used rather glibly so far, 'science'. We have discussed science as a collection of methods; that is, how facts are acquired and hypotheses tested in the social and biological sciences. But there is more to science than the methods. It is a word that carries many other meanings.

    ☐   Think of at least two other meanings of the term 'science'.

    ■   First, as well as a collection of methods, 'science' is often taken to refer to the body of facts, laws, theories and relationships concerning real phenomena which the methods of science have apparently revealed to be true statements about the world. Second, 'science' is taken to mean the body of 'scientists' and the set of social institutions in which they participate: the journals, books, laboratories, professional societies and academies through which individuals and the work they do are given currency and legitimacy.

Yet the central question about scientific knowledge — and one that produces much debate among philosophers, and much confusion among scientists and non-scientists alike — concerns the *status* of scientific knowledge. What science — natural or social — *says* the world is like, is not identical to the world itself. Observations, data and experiments are all designed to test particular theories, or are planned with a particular model in mind.

The methodology of the social sciences

If relating observations and facts to theories about those observations is hard enough in biology, it is still harder in the social sciences. Consider, for example, how the methods discussed in Chapters 7–10 might be applied to running a large NHS hospital. Everyone has an interest in how it is run — its staff, obviously, but also all citizens, as taxpayers and potential patients.

    ☐   What sorts of criteria might be useful in assessing whether the hospital is well run?

    ■   Many different criteria may have occurred to you, for example: Is the patient treated politely? Is money spent wisely or extravagantly? Are the staff properly trained? Do they actually improve the patient's condition?

Putting this more generally, there are three principal criteria by which the hospital might be assessed: is it *effective*; is it *efficient*; is it *humane*? Let us examine each of these in a little more detail.

    ☐   What sorts of things should one look at to assess the hospital's effectiveness?

    ■   These questions are likely to be of particular interest. How often do the patients die (the fatality rate)? Do the treatments actually work? Or do they even harm some patients (e.g. do patients pick up infections, or are they damaged by drugs that are prescribed)?

    ☐   What aspects of the hospital need examination if one is to judge its efficiency?

    ■   There are many things to look at here. First there are the hospital's costs — salaries, maintenance bills and expenditure on new buildings and equipment. One must also examine its buying policies — does it get its drugs as cheaply as it could? How are important decisions made? Is all the appropriate information to hand? Most importantly, would it be possible to attain a higher level of effectiveness with the same amount of resources, or the same level of effectiveness with fewer resources, by altering working practices or by rearranging the equipment and staffing of the hospital?

    ☐   What would count as evidence of humanity?

    ■   Obviously, the way patients are treated is important. Are the staff polite and friendly? Do patients get all the necessary information? Is special care taken to ensure that patients do not suffer unnecessary fears or pain? And how are the staff themselves treated? Do the laundry workers and the junior doctors get a fair deal?

There is, then, a long list of important criteria that, ideally, the hospital should meet. One could conduct research into these using the methods that were discussed earlier. But a theory of human behaviour is also needed to enable one both to interpret the findings and to suggest how the hospital might be made more efficient, more effective or more humane.

There are many theories of human social behaviour, but they all start from one of two broad premises: either that individual people's interests tend to generate a harmonious society; or that they tend to generate a society of conflict. Do all hospital personnel work together as a team, or are the interests of nurses different from those of doctors and cleaners? Are the interests of hospital staff the same as those of hospital patients? Harmony or conflict? The first type of theory is known as *functionalism*, the second, simply, as *conflict theory*.

Functionalism sees the staff and patients of a hospital as sharing a common set of values and goals. There are differences between them in the tasks they have to perform but each is valued by the other and each task serves an important need, whether of an individual or the group as a whole. So closely are staff and patients intertwined that when problems arise peace and harmony are soon restored.

Conflict theory claims that there are irreconcilable differences between the interests, say of hospital cleaners needing a living wage, a limited number of hours of work a week and well-defined conditions of service, and those of doctors, patients or administrators. Conflict theory sees ideas of peace and harmony merely as propaganda dished out by the hospital elite in order to retain their positions in the hierarchy of power, prestige and income. Sometimes peace may appear to reign in the hospital but this is a momentary illusion, for occasionally the weak give up their struggle, disheartened by their position or temporarily blinded by current propaganda.

It is, of course, an oversimplification to draw such a sharp distinction between functionalism and conflict theory. Functionalists do admit the existence of conflict; but they often see this, in its turn, as functional for the hospital. Likewise, conflict theorists hold a more subtle view of the nature of conflict than that portrayed here. They often stress the incompatability of *group* interests, rather than the force or cunning of the individual. Both positions are explored in more detail elsewhere; for the moment you should merely note that not all conflict theorists believe in the inevitability of extreme conflict. Many argue that this occurs only under *certain* conditions. Depending on how the hospital is organised, it will be either full of conflict, or harmonious.

☐ How should a hospital be run to ensure that everyone's needs are satisfied? Can you think of any political or economic theories as to how this might be accomplished?

■ One major theory of how to do this is socialism, which argues that the hospital should be run collectively, with the staff and patients sharing power. By contrast, the theory of neo-classical economics argues that individual needs are satisfied only when every individual can bargain for precisely what they want. To this end hospital care should be paid for individually, hospitals should compete with one another and no group of staff should have a monopoly. To this the socialists respond that such individual bargaining works only when every individual has equal resources with which to bargain — something that will not be true of laundry workers or the chronically ill.

We have now advanced quite a way towards working out how to run a good hospital. Criteria — efficiency, effectiveness and humanity — have been specified, a variety of methods have been devised to check these criteria are being met and the main theories of how hospitals work or might be made to work better have just been considered. There is, however, a major flaw in our analysis. The hospital has been considered as if it stood *alone*, completely separate from the rest of the social world.

☐ What are some of the ways in which the staff of the hospital might be affected by the following social institutions: age, class, gender, ethnicity, government, trade unions, the law, the economy, and other societies?

■ These are obviously all complex issues, but you should have come up with at least some of the following: *age* — hospitals have special facilities and staff for certain age-groups, such as children and the elderly; *class* — there is a definite social class hierarchy within British hospitals, doctors in class I, nurses in class II, secretaries in class III, and so on; *gender* — there is also a gender hierarchy within the hospital: the most senior staff, the doctors, tend to be men, whereas many of the more junior staff, such as nurses and cleaners, tend to be women; *ethnicity* — there is also a clear ethnic hierarchy within the hospital: the lowlier the staff, the more likely they are to be of New Commonwealth origin; *government* — the hospital is not self-governing: its finances and many of its priorities are determined by the local health authority, by the civil service and ultimately by the ministers of a particular political party which in its turn is subject to re-election; *trade unions* — most of the staff of the hospital, including doctors and nurses, will belong to trade unions, each of which is seeking better pay and working conditions; the *law* — many of the hospital's activities are subject to wider laws, from the terms of employment of its staff to the conditions under which they may perform abortions; the *economy* — the health service, of which the hospital is a part, is the largest employer in Britain, and buys an enormous quantity of drugs, equipment, bedding and so forth from other sectors of industry; *other societies* —

many hospital staff are likely to have been trained in other countries, and all of them use knowledge and goods that were created in other societies.

In thinking about this external framework within which the hospital is embedded one finds once again competing functionalist and conflict theories; the one holding that all these different parts, of which the hospital is merely one, form a harmonious sytem, the other seeing.them as locked in fierce competition.

The same two theories are also used to explain another important feature of the hospital and its environment. As we have seen, staff and patients each belong to a series of hierarchies: age, gender, ethnicity, class, and the like. Such hierarchies are normally known by social scientists as *stratification systems*. The word stratification is a metaphor borrowed from geology. There it refers to the way in which layers of different sorts of rock are piled one on top of another to form different 'strata'. Social science applies this to social as well as geological formations, for just about every aspect of human life appears to be stratified in one way or another.

Although stratification is universal, different sorts of stratification get more or less prominence in different types of society. For example, age and gender stratification systems appear to be universal, whereas stratification into 'social classes' is characteristic of large, wealthy, complex societies. Functionalists see hierarchies in the hospital, or elsewhere, as a natural product of the need to organise social life efficiently. Society has need of this or that capacity, and those with more of the relevant talents go to the top, those with fewer to the bottom. Conflict theory argues that the real explanation is power. Those who have power use this to exploit those who do not.

So what the study of the hospital encompasses is now reasonably clear. There are criteria by which to judge it — efficiency, effectiveness and humanity. There are two possible theories of how hospitals might work — functionalism and conflict theory. The way in which the hospital is embedded in a wider world must also be considered. But what sorts of methods should be used in the investigation? In previous chapters of this book both numerical and qualitative methods have been reviewed. What might each contribute to the study? Let us take just one aspect of the hospital and consider the methodological question in more detail.

One of the most controversial public debates over Britain's National Health Service concerns doctors' and nurses' wages — their level, their difference and the ways in which they are determined.

☐ If one wanted to research this question of wages, for which topics would numerical methods be needed and for which topics would qualitative?

■ Numerical methods would be needed to describe the precise differences in doctors' and nurses' wages, how they have changed relative to each other over time and their relation to inflation and to the wages in other comparable occupations. But we also need information on matters such as the relationship of each group of staff to the political parties (in Britain, does the Conservative Party favour the doctors and Labour the nurses?), the historical development of the medical monopoly and the relations between men and women in our society. These topics need qualitative as well as numerical investigation.

The two methods are locked in an endless cycle, each throwing up new problems for the other to solve, each casting light on matters that the other has thus far neglected. Qualitative researchers have a tendency to roam; their numerical colleagues focus on a single topic and count. Each has its advantages as a method for studying the social complexities of health and disease.

Levels of analysis and levels of explanation: race and ethnicity

In the discussion of the hospital we have tried to show how contrasting theories and methods endeavour to explain a complex social structure. But how do these different types of social explanation relate to the types of biological explanation we discussed in the first part of the chapter? We have emphasised that we are committed to the unity of knowledge and explanation, yet clearly there remain formidable difficulties in the way of providing comprehensive causal explanations. Perhaps one could just accept that there may be only one world, but many different ways of describing it? After all, we are trying to describe the world not just in order to understand it, but in order to intervene directly in its workings. As you saw in the case of the hospital, very little biological knowledge is necessary to evaluate whether the hospital is efficient, effective or humane.

Sometimes attempts to unify biological and social understanding can even confuse matters. Take one example: that of race and ethnicity. In everyday language, people use the word 'race' very loosely. They speak of white or black 'races', distinguishing people by skin colour, or of the Jewish 'race', distinguishing by culture, and even English, Irish, Scottish and Welsh 'races', distinguishing by nationality. But what does the term 'race' mean? Locked away in these uses of the word is the assumption that underlying the *social* label is a *biological* basis, that there are biologically distinguishing features that separate one 'race' from another. This belief, and this use of the word 'race', has deep roots in British cultural history. It dominated the thinking of much nineteenth- and early twentieth-century anthropology, and reached its most extreme form in Nazi theory, in which 'races' were subdivided still further: for example, the Europeans into Aryan, Nordic and Mediterranean 'types' and *Untermenschen* ('subhumans') like 'Slavs' and 'Jews'.

However, these popular uses of the word 'race' have little, if anything, to do with biology. For biologists, 'race' is a technical term, which may apply to all species*. A race is defined biologically as a population, a subset of a species, within which there is a free exchange of genes by interbreeding, and which may be distinguished from other populations by some common and heritable attribute. Normally such a racial group is formed when there is a barrier over many generations to breeding with other groups.

In the early days of the study of human 'races', a century ago, much attention was devoted to readily observable physical differences, for instance, in skin or hair colour or bodily physique. However, geneticists today recognise that such studies may be very misleading. Instead, they attempt to measure directly the genes present in particular human groups. Many genes are known to exist in alternative forms, called *alleles*. (For instance, a person's blood group, A, B, O or whatever, is determined by which of a particular set of alleles of the genes for the blood group proteins they have. Different people have different alleles, hence different blood groups.) One can then study the frequency with which a particular allele occurs in any given group. A distinct human 'race', in the biological sense, would exist if the frequency with which a particular allele occurred in that group was very different from the frequency with which it occurred in another.

There are races in animal populations, but are there in humans? When allele frequencies are measured in human populations that are *socially* defined as races (for instance, 'English', 'Jews', 'Blacks'), it turns out that for nearly all the genes studied the differences between individuals of different 'races' are no greater than for individuals of the same 'race'. *Well over 94 per cent of all the differences are found within a given 'race' rather than between 'races'.* This means that, genetically, a white English individual is likely to be just as similar to or different from his white neighbour as he is to a Caribbean or Asian neighbour.

Of course, there are genetic differences between individuals; everyone, except identical twins, is genetically unique. But classifying the genetic uniqueness 'racially' only confuses the issue. Differences in the distribution of

particular alleles may occur between regions (e.g. between north and south Wales) or even close villages. Yet no one would think of classifying these as 'racial' differences. (Nor is 'racial purity' a meaningful concept, as can be seen by a study of allele frequency in samples of Jews and their non-Jewish neighbours. *Genetically*, for the alleles studied, Polish Jews resemble their Catholic neighbours more than they do, say, Spanish Jews.)

As a final example, consider the American population. This derives from extensive interbreeding between European, Asian, African and native American Indian peoples and represents a mixture of the genes from people of all these groups. Today, within America, a person is defined as Black or White on the basis of skin colour, yet this is determined by only a very small number of genes. A 'White' person may have many more genes deriving from his or her African ancestors than a neighbouring 'Black' — but *not* have the tiny number of genes responsible for black skin colour!

It is as a result of observations like these that modern biology is coming to discard the concept of 'race' as having any relevance to the study of human populations. This means that if social scientists use the term 'race' it has a meaning quite different from that which biologists might give it. This is one of the reasons why social scientists these days tend to talk about *ethnicity* rather than race. At least one reason is that ethnicity, that is, the ascription of an individual to a group based on a complex of factors such as religion, culture and natural origin, ought to be easier to measure, should we want to do so. Many people argue, for instance, that there is a need for information on ethnic groupings in Britain. How might one set about obtaining this information?

Several official government surveys already make classifications according to 'race' or 'ethnic origin', but it is not clear what exactly they are measuring. In one such survey, the General Household Survey, interviewers were asked to classify people as 'white' or 'coloured' subjectively, by observing their skin colour alone. Other surveys ask respondents to choose how to describe themselves from a list of categories such as West Indian or Bengali. Perhaps the most widely used measure is based on information from the census on the 'place of birth of respondent' and (from the 1971 census) the 'birth place of parents'. Estimates have been made from this data of the number of people from the 'New Commonwealth' countries living in Britain (the so-called 'coloured' population). However, this question turned out to be unsatisfactory.

☐ Can you suggest some reasons why this might have been so?
■ As a measure of 'ethnic' or 'cultural' origin categories based on place of birth are very crude. Some

---

* A species is a group of living organisms capable of interbreeding but isolated reproductively from other such groups. Thus retrievers and cocker spaniels are members of the same species, as they can interbreed. Dogs and cats are examples of two separate species.

'white' people born overseas to British parents were difficult to identify. Some people did not know the place of birth of their parents. Even assuming that what was wanted was 'colour', some 'coloured' people were not identified by the question as they and their parents were born in Britain.

Because of the inadequacy of existing data on ethnicity the Office of Population Censuses and Surveys began in 1974 to devise an 'ethnic question' to be included in the 1981 census. The actual question finally proposed and the controversy that surrounded it illustrate the considerable difficulties involved in devising a measure of ethnicity. The question involved a whole range of different interpretations of ethnicity. It confused categories of skin colour, geographical origin, cultural/ethnic origin and religion. (For example, people were asked to describe themselves as being of one or other of the following races or ethnic origins: White, West Indian, African, Arab, Turkish, Chinese, Indian, Pakistani, Bangladeshi or Sri Lankan.) It is not at all clear what the census office meant by race or ethnic groups. Many people argued that ethnicity was essentially a subjective phenomenon and that the question did not allow for this. British-born black people for example were not able to define themselves as 'British', though they might have felt themselves to be so. The question was also widely seen to be discriminatory.

- ☐ Can you suggest some reasons for this criticism?
- ■ The question divides the population into 'white'

and others. No attempt was made to distinguish between different white ethnic groups.

Similarly, no attempt was made to identify religion other than those prevalent in (but by no means restricted to) the Indian subcontinent.

The controversy surrounding the development of this question also highlighted fears among some ethnic minority communities that 'ethnic' information might be misused. This was a particularly sensitive issue as concern was growing about the possibility of repatriation in the light of a new nationality bill. The more general issue of privacy and confidentiality was also an important topic in the debate.

The growing support for the collection of 'ethnic' data has therefore been paralleled by growing opposition to it on the grounds that it is racist and discriminatory to classify people according to skin colour or social divisions that many believe should not exist. However, there is a dilemma, for although one might accept that they should not exist, such 'divisions' have a very real impact on the people involved. It has been demonstrated, for instance, that discrimination is most often based purely on skin colour rather than on ethnicity or race. In the event no question on ethnicity was included in the census. It is possible that information on the circumstances and needs of ethnic minority groups can be collected sensitively on a smaller scale than the census provides for. But if national data on ethnicity are to be collected, it would seem that the nature of the information that is required should be clarified, and non-discriminatory questions devised.

Objectives for Chapter 11

When you have studied this chapter, you should be able to:

11.1 Distinguish between different meanings of 'science', and between facts and theories.

11.2 Define and give examples of the use of three types of causal explanation of health and disease: reductionist, holistic, and temporal; and describe the relationships between them.

11.3 Describe and exemplify functionalist and conflict theories of social structure and social change in the context of health and disease.

11.4 Understand the difficulties in the use of the terms 'race' and 'ethnicity' and distinguish between social and biological meanings of the word 'race'.

Questions for Chapter 11

1 (*Objective 11.1*) Which of the several senses of the word 'science' is being used in each of the following statements?

(i) 'More money needed for medical science', says Ministry of Health.

(ii) Science has proved that one type of diabetes is caused by a deficiency of insulin production in the sufferer.

(iii) It is scientifically true to say that insulin is a protein produced in the pancreas.

2 (*Objective 11.2*) Offer (a) a reductionist, (b) a holistic and (c) a temporal explanation of Mr Lawson's diabetes.

3 (*Objective 11.1*) Which of the following statements is a fact, and which is a theory about diabetes?

(a) Diabetes is the name given to a disease characterised by a high level of blood sugar and the presence of sugar in the urine.

(b) Diabetes is caused by a combination of dietary effects and a genetic propensity to the disorder.

(c) Insulin is a protein secreted by particular cells of the pancreas.

(d) Lack of insulin causes diabetes as insulin is involved in the regulation of sugar metabolism in the muscle and liver.

4 (*Objective 11.3*) Which of the following situations fits either functionalist or conflict theories?

(a) The government of a country with a state-run health system decides to privatise the hospital service.

(b) As a result, large sections of the staff go on strike.

(c) There is a large press and television campaign against the strikers, and eventually they return to work.

(d) In the end some hospitals are privatised, others are run cooperatively.

5 (*Objective 11.4*) Which of the following is a statement about ethnicity and which is a statement that might relate to a biologically defined group or race?

(a) Marriages between cousins tend to be frequent in Asian families living in England.

(b) Jews living in England whose families have originated from Eastern Europe are more liable to be affected by Tay-Sachs disease, a progressive genetic disorder, than non-Jewish, white people born in England and Wales.

(c) Scots are proverbially mean.

(d) In Britain today, children of Asian origin tend on average to get better grades in O and A levels than children of Caribbean origin.

12
Understanding and changing the world

So far, we have given a rather static picture of the world. But time is central to the whole of life; we are in a constant process of change. Diabetes used to be a chronic disease but one of relatively short duration. Most of its victims did not live long. It is now, thanks to insulin, a disease primarily of long-term complications. These effects are the by-product of human intervention. So too is the most dramatic short-term problem that diabetics now suffer. The hypoglycaemic attack, caused by too little sugar in the blood, is a direct product of insulin therapy.

Minkowski and Banting, and those who applied their work, have created the modern form of diabetes. This form will go on changing. New techniques for achieving better control will create new forms of diabetes. Likewise, as diabetes is modified, so it modifies us. Human intervention in disease changes the average genetic composition of the population. Moreover, the changing diet of the industrial world and the fact that diabetics now live longer both produce an increased proportion of diabetes sufferers in the population. Given the expansion of the diabetic population, relevant sections of the medical, food and drug industries expand in their turn.

Human society thus not only changes fast but in extremely complex ways. It is only 10 000 years since the first 'agricultural revolution'; the Industrial Revolution is a mere 200 years old and has, perhaps, barely begun.

How can these extraordinary historical changes be explained? The functionalist theory of history accounts for the differences between tribal and industrialised societies by pointing to the progressive development of the *division of labour*. Over time the execution of those tasks vital to the fulfilment of human needs has been enormously improved by individuals coming to specialise in particular activities, or parts of those activities. However, there is also a conflict version. This points to the following facts: some people benefit from changes more than others; some get the opportunity to change, others do not; and some resist change and have it forced upon them. Societies are divided by disparities in wealth, status and power. These disparities separate social classes, genders and ethnic groups. Change comes about, therefore, as the product of human struggle.

Let us now apply the two theories to something we have touched on in the context of Snow's recognition of the causes of cholera. The nineteenth-century public health movement involved major changes in sanitation, in bacteriology, in the understanding of the social distribution of disease and in public knowledge about the way to combat disease.

☐ How would functionalist theory explain these changes?

■ Functionalists would argue that by the nineteenth century, new sorts of occupation were developing on the basis of new forms of knowledge. Engineers had developed the capacity for major sanitation schemes. The new disciplines of statistics and social science had begun to explore the social and geographical distribution of disease. The new science of bacteriology, created by people such as Pasteur, was developing germ theory. Finally, reformers such as Florence Nightingale, and a new breed of nurse, the health visitor, were campaigning for cleanliness.

A conflict explanation of the same events would cover some of the following points: (a) the political struggles of the working-classes and Irish immigrants who suffered most from these diseases; (b) the feminist movement fighting for women's rights; (c) conflict between *laissez-faire* and state-interventionist approaches to the solution of social problems; (d) the professional struggle for the control of the medical arena, between doctors on the one hand and engineers, statisticians and social scientists on the other.

In whatever way history is explained, *progress* in certain areas is undeniable. Not very long ago, infectious disease was one of the greatest terrors of the Western world. It is no longer. Changes such as this have led to a distinct shift in the modern world-view. Over the last few centuries Western society has developed a natural as opposed to a super-natural view of the world. This has radically changed the way in which both history and our place in that history are viewed. Because this new view of progress informs nearly every aspect of our thinking about health and disease, it deserves close inspection.

In previous ages, when people thought about their ideas of health, they looked to the past, the Golden Age. When they looked to the future they saw nothing but a continuation of present misery: life was hard and not much could be expected from it. Famine and pestilence were the regular lot of humanity. That change occurred could not be denied. But the standard theory of history was essentially cyclical. New empires rose, shattering the old, only to be replaced, in their turn, by still newer powers. The medieval image of history was the Wheel of Fortune, eternally rising, only to fall again to where it had begun. Human aspiration was either comic or tragic, pride going before a fall.

By the end of the eighteenth century, all this had begun to change. Economic growth, coupled with the new sciences, led to the hope that humanity could escape from the Wheel of Fortune, could rise without falling. This was the age of Enlightenment, an age with whose hopes we still live. To the believer in enlightenment, science, both natural and social, at last permits people to shape their own destiny — if it is used wisely and well. Disease may be conquered, or at least tamed.

Such is the most optimistic view. Not everyone has shared it. The idea of progress has been qualified in three important ways. Anthropologists have shown that the break with the past is not complete; tribal and industrial societies still have many things in common. Recent history has shown that the new knowledge is not neutral; it has evil as well as good purposes; it might indeed destroy us all. Physics has led to the hydrogen bomb, medical science to biological warfare. Even if done with the best of intentions, the application of new knowledge can sometimes increase disease and suffering, not reduce it. Thalidomide is a classic modern example. Both natural and social scientists have become aware of the limitations of their knowledge and of the unintended consequences of human intervention. We know enough to intervene in history; we cannot always predict the results of intervention. We have not escaped entirely from the Wheel of Fortune.

These doubts about progress should make us all pause. They should not inhibit all further intervention. Bismarck, the Iron Chancellor, the creator of the nineteenth-century German state as well as the founder of state health insurance, once remarked that, though people are never in full control of events, occasionally they are in a position to deflect them to their advantage. In other words, if we get our timing and analysis right, we can sometimes steer things in the direction we prefer. This book is about how we might learn to do this better in health and disease.

References
and
further
reading

References

ASHER, RICHARD   (1972) *Talking Sense*, Pitman Medical.

BEESON, PAUL B.   (1977) The development of clinical knowledge, with a few words about targeted vs. basic research, *Journal of the American Medical Association*, 237, No. 20 (May 16), pp. 2209–12.

BEISCHER, N. A., EVANS, J. H. and TOWNSEND, L.   (1979) Studies of prolonged pregnancy. I The incidence of prolonged pregnancy, *American Journal of Obstetrics and Gynecology*, 103, pp. 476–82.

BLACK, NICK, BOSWELL, DAVID, GRAY, ALASTAIR, MURPHY, SEAN and POPAY, JENNY (eds) (1984) *Health and Disease: A Reader*, The Open University Press. The Course Reader.

BOSK, CHARLES   (1979) *Forgive and Remember: Managing Medical Failure*, University of Chicago Press.

BULGAKOV, MIKHAIL   (1975) The steel windpipe, in his *A Country Doctor's Notebook*, trans. Michael Glenny, Collins and Harvill (first published in 1927)

CARTWRIGHT, A. and BOWLING, A.   (1982) *Life After Death: A Study of the Elderly Widowed*, Tavistock.

DEPARTMENT OF EMPLOYMENT   (1980) *New Earnings Survey 1980, Part A*, HMSO.

DEPARTMENT OF HEALTH AND SOCIAL SECURITY   (1976) *Prevention and Health: Everybody's Business*, HMSO.

DEUTSCHER, IRWIN   (1969) Looking backwards: case studies in the progress of social methodology, *American Sociologist*, 4, pp. 35–41.

ENGELHARDT JR, H. TRISTRAM   (1981) Clinical judgment, *Metamedicine*, 2, pp. 301–17.

FOX, A. J. and GOLDBLATT, P. D.   (1982) *Longitudinal Study: Socio-demographic Mortality Differentials 1971–75*, HMSO.

JAMES, N., LAURENCE, K. M. and MILLER, M.   (1980) Diet as a factor in the aetiology of neural tube malformations, *Zeitschrift für Kinderchirurgie*, 31, pp. 302–7.

KING, LESTER S.   (1954) What is disease?, *Philosophy of Science*, 21, pp. 193–203.

KINSEY, ALFRED *et al.*,   (1948) *Sexual Behavior in the Human Male*, W. B. Saunders, Philadelphia.

KINSEY, ALFRED *et al.*,   (1953) *Sexual Behavior in the Human Female*, W. B. Saunders, Philadelphia.

LAURENCE, K. M., CAMPBELL, H. and JAMES, N.   (1983) The role of improvement in the maternal diet and preconceptional folic acid supplementation in the prevention of neural tube defects, in Dobbing, J (ed.) (1983) *Prevention of Spina Bifida and Other Neural Tube Defects*, Academic Press.

LAURENCE, K. M., JAMES, N., MILLER, M. and CAMPBELL, H.   (1980) Increased risk of recurrence of pregnancies complicated by foetal neural tube defects in mothers receiving poor diets, and possible benefits of dietary counselling, *British Medical Journal*, 281, pp. 1592–4.

LAURENCE, K. M., JAMES, NANSI, MILLER, MARY, TENNANT, G. B. and CAMPBELL, H.   (1981) Double-blind randomised controlled trial of folate treatment before conception to prevent recurrence of neural-tube defects, *British Medical Journal*, 282, pp. 1509–11; in the Course Reader.

MELBIN, MURRAY   (1969) Behaviour rhythms in mental hospitals, *American Journal of Sociology*, 74(6), pp. 650–665.

MILLMAN, MARCIA (1978) *The Unkindest Cut: Life in the Backrooms of Medicine*, Morrow, New York.

OPCS (1978) *Occupational Mortality: The Registrar General's Decennial Supplement for England and Wales 1970–72*, Series DS, No. 1, HMSO.

OPCS (1981) *Population Estimates, England and Wales 1980*, Series PP1, No. 5, HMSO.

OPCS (1982a) *Birth Statistics 1980, England and Wales*, Series FM1, No. 7, HMSO.

OPCS (1982b) *Mortality Statistics; Childhood, England and Wales 1980*, Series DH3, No. 8, HMSO.

OPCS (1982c) *Mortality Statistics: Area, England and Wales 1980*, Series DH5, No. 7, HMSO.

OPCS (1982d) *Mortality Statistics: Cause, England and Wales 1980*, Series DH2, No. 7, HMSO.

OPCS (1982e) *Mortality Statistics, Perinatal and Infant: Social and Biological Factors. England and Wales 1978, 1979*, Series DH3, No. 7, HMSO.

POSNER, TINA (1977) Magical elements in orthodox medicine, in Dingwall, R. *et al.* (eds) (1977) *Health Care and Health Knowledge*, Croom-Helm; in the Course Reader.

RADICAL STATISTICS HEALTH GROUP (1976) *Whose Priorities?* Radical Statistics.

REGISTRAR GENERAL SCOTLAND (1982) *Annual Report for 1980*, HMSO.

SMITHELLS, R. W., SHEPPARD, S., SCHORAH, C. J., SELLER, M. J., NEVIN, N. C., HARRIS, R., READ, A. P. and FIELDING, D. W. (1980) Possible prevention of neural tube defects by periconceptional vitamin supplementation, *The Lancet*, i, pp. 339–40; in the Course Reader.

Social Trends (1975) HMSO.

STRONG, P. M. (1979) *The Ceremonial Order of the Clinic*, Routledge and Kegan Paul.

TATTERSALL, R. B. and JACKSON, J. G. L. (1982) Social and emotional complications of diabetes, in Keen, H. and Jarret, J. (1982) *Complications of Diabetes*, 2nd edn, Edward Arnold.

The Concise Oxford Dictionary of Current English (1976) 6th edn, Oxford University Press.

The Lancet (1980), July 26th, p. 189.

THE OPEN UNIVERSITY (1983) MDST 242 *Statistics in Society*, Unit C3 *Is My Child Normal?*, The Open University Press.

THE REGISTRAR GENERAL (1970) *Classification of Occupations*, cited in Reid, I. (1981) *Social Class Differences in Britain*, 2nd edn, Grant McIntyre.

UNITED NATIONS (1977) *UN Demographic Year Book, 1977*, United Nations, New York.

UNITED NATIONS (1980) *UN Demographic Year Book, 1980*, United Nations, New York.

VAN DEN BERG, JAN H. (1981) *The Psychology of the Sickbed*, Humanities Press, New Jersey.

WATSON, J. D. and CRICK, F. H. C. (1953) A structure for DNA, *Nature*, **171**, pp. 736–8.

WILKINSON, D. G. (1981) Psychiatric aspects of diabetes mellitus, *British Journal of Psychiatry*, **138**, pp. 1–9.

Further reading

ASHER, RICHARD (1972) *Talking Sense*, Pitman Medical.
This collection of papers by Richard Asher offers a clinician's view of the world of health, disease and medicine. Often amusing, always entertaining and provocative, the essays discuss the actual experience of practising medicine — those aspects that more formal accounts fail to mention. Though there are many accounts of what patients think of doctors, this is a rare example of the reverse.

BARKER, D. J. P. and ROSE, G. (1984) *Epidemiology in Medical Practice*, 3rd edn, Churchill Livingstone.
This is a short, introductory textbook of epidemiology. It is divided into three sections: the methods used to describe the distribution of disease in populations; the methods used to discover the causes of disease; and those aspects of health care that require an understanding of epidemiology — screening, prognosis, epidemics and the evaluation of medical services.

HAMMERSLEY, M. and ATKINSON, P. (1983) *Ethnography: Principles in Practice*, Tavistock.
A major review of some qualitative methods and studies.

MCCALL, G. J. and SIMMONS, J. L. (eds) (1969) *Issues in Participant Observation: A Text and Reader*, Addison-Wesley, Massachusetts.
A classic collection of articles.

MARSH, C. (1982) *The Survey Method*, George Allen & Unwin.
A good introduction to the use of questionnaires.

Statistics

Statistics published by Government departments and other institutions play a very important role in the study of health and disease. However, if you have ever tried to trace a particular piece of information which you think has been published, you will realise that it is not always easy to find what you want. It is not possible to provide you with a guide to sources of published health statistics. Some other places you might look for such a guide are as follows:

RADICAL STATISTICS HEALTH GROUP (1981) *An Unofficial Guide to Official Health Statistics*, Radical Statistics, c/o BSSRS, 9 Poland Street, London, W1. A brief, clear, critical guide to Government health statistics. Recommended.

Two volumes in the Social Science Research Council/Royal Statistical Society's series of *Reviews of United Kingdom Statistical Sources* are useful as they are full, critical guides to the areas they cover (though the first of them is somewhat out of date).

ALDERSON, M. R. (1973) Central Government Routine Health Statistics, in Volume II of *Reviews of United Kingdom Statistical Sources*, Heinemann Educational Books.

ALDERSON, M. R. and DOWIE, R. (1979) Health Surveys and Related Studies, in Volume IX of *Reviews of United Kingdom Statistical Sources*, Pergamon Press.

Acknowledgements

Grateful acknowledgement is made to the following sources for material used in this book:

Tables
Table 6.1 adapted from N. James *et al.* in J. Dobbing (ed.) *Prevention of Spina Bifida and other Neural Tube Defects*, Academic Press Inc. (London) Ltd, 1983.

Figures
Frontispiece and Figure 3.2 courtesy of The Wellcome Institute; *Figure 3.1* courtesy of the British Museum; *Figure 3.3 (a–d)* courtesy of Scanning Unit, Royal Post Graduate School, Hammersmith Hospital; *Figure 4.15* from *Occupational Mortality: The Registrar General's Decennial Supplement for England and Wales 1970–72*, 1978, reproduced by permission of the Controller of HMSO; *Figure 5.1* courtesy of The Wellcome Institute; *Figure 5.5* Crown copyright, reproduced by permission of the Controller of HMSO; *Figure 5.6* from DHSS, *Prevention and Health: Everybody's Business*, 1976, reproduced by permission of the Controller of HMSO; *Figure 5.7* from Radical Statistics Health Group, *Whose Priorities?*, 1976, reproduced by permission of Radical Statistics.

Answers to self-assessment questions

Chapter 2

1 The answers are: (a) disease; (b) symptom; (c) sign; (d) symptom; (e) sign; (f) disease.

2 You may have guessed from the phrasing of the question and the discussion in the text that what used to be described as myocardial degeneration is now usually classified as coronary heart disease. Thus some of the apparent rise in the numbers of deaths from the latter will simply reflect a change in the categorisation of diseases. This alteration reflects changes in the theoretical interests of medicine — from the pathological appearance of the heart after death to the patency of the blood vessels supplying the heart (coronary arteries), which can be demonstrated using sophisticated modern technology.

3 If you found this question hard to answer then you probably understand the difficulties of defining 'health' and 'disease'. This example illustrates how it is possible to feel healthy and yet harbour a disease. Similarly, one may feel unwell, even though doctors will claim there is no disease present.

4 The case series. If a doctor sees several people suffering from the rash, and they have all used the new washing powder, then it is likely that the rash and the use of the powder are causally related. However, if the doctor studies only one person with the rash (a case-study approach) it is unlikely that the association with the washing powder will be spotted. This is because both skin rashes and exposure to all sorts of substances (such as washing powders) are common occurrences (rather like sparrows on a bird-table!).

Chapter 3

1 There are several described, but you might have chosen: (i) *observation* — dogs that have had their pancreas removed develop diabetes mellitus; (ii) *hypothesis* — there is a substance normally present in pancreatic extract which is absent in diabetics; (iii) *testing the hypothesis* — injections of extracts of pancreatic juice alleviate the symptoms of diabetes in dogs and humans.

2 (a) Some examples are: (i) *body fluid analysis* — the discovery of high levels of sugar in blood and urine; (ii) *genetic studies* — looking at the distribution of diabetes within and between families; (iii) *post-mortem studies* — you might have thought of examining the pancreas from people who have died from diabetes, although we did not mention this. (Such an examination may show a characteristic loss of particular cell types involved in insulin production.)

(b) None of these studies would be able to tell you exactly how insulin acted at the cellular level. Indeed, they could not tell you about insulin at all — all you could deduce was that there is an inherited tendency to suffer diabetes, which is characterised by high sugar levels in blood and urine, and that in diabetes, some cells of the pancreas seem to be abnormal or absent. But this could be a *consequence* rather than a *cause* of the disease.

3 (a) You might have chosen from any of the following levels of analysis: (i) *intact organism* — an injection of insulin controls the level of blood sugar in the circulation; (ii) *slice of liver or muscle tissue* — incubation in solution containing insulin shows that the amount of sugar taken up by the slice depends on the amount of insulin in the surrounding medium; (iii) *preparation of broken-up cells* — study of this shows insulin does not affect the metabolism of sugar and therefore must affect the *uptake* of the sugar into the cells; (iv) *molecular level* — the purification of insulin shows it to be a protein molecule present in pancreatic juice.

(b) Each level of analysis is necessary because, for instance, a study at the level of the intact organism could never tell you that insulin was a protein which can be purified and preserved in a stable form available to diabetics to treat themselves with. A study of the chemistry of insulin alone could never demonstrate that it was effective in the treatment of diabetes, nor reveal just how it works by enabling sugar to enter the cell.

4 Among other things you could not know what it *felt* like to suffer diabetes from animal models. You could not be sure of the genetic involvement in human diabetes, as it is

clearly not a simple genetic disorder. You could not discover the role of changing environmental circumstances in diabetes except very simple ones such as diet, or the role of occupation. And you could not predict the psychological and social consequences of a therapeutic regime that makes sufferers dependent for the rest of their lives on regular injections of insulin.

Chapter 4

1 The mean is:

$$\frac{\text{total}}{\text{size}} = \frac{683}{8} = 85.375.$$

2 (a) The rate per thousand is:

$$\frac{1\,479}{89\,397} \times 1\,000 = 16.5.$$

(b) The PNMR increases steadily as we go from social class I to social class V. Perinatal mortality is far more of a problem in the families of unskilled manual workers than in the families of professional men.

3 (a) The row percentages for Table 4.7 are set out in Table 4.7 (answers at the foot of this page).

(b) Compared with Aylesbury Vale, Milton Keynes has a younger population. In particular, Milton Keynes has proportionately far more younger adults (20–39) and far fewer middle-aged people (40–64) than Aylesbury Vale. Milton Keynes also has fewer elderly people and more teenagers and children.

4 (a) The relationship is positive, because the points on the scatter diagram slope upwards from left to right.

(b) The higher the smoking ratio in an occupational group the higher is the standardised mortality ratio for lung· cancer. So, in terms of the meanings given to these quantities in the question, the more the men in an occupational group smoke, the more of them will die from lung cancer.

(c) No. There is nothing *in these data* to show the relationship is causal. (But there are many more data available on the link between smoking and disease!)

(d) The data are cross-sectional. They were collected by studying a whole population over a short period of time, rather than by following up individuals over a long time and examining changes over time.

Chapter 5

1 An epidemiologist would be interested in all of these except, possibly, (iii). That is, because epidemiology is the study of health and disease in populations, (i), (ii) and (iv) are of interest. But Mr Lawson's case *in itself* would not be studied in epidemiology. However, an epidemiologist might well be interested in a systematic comparison of a group of people that *included* Mr Lawson with some other group, and Mr Lawson's diagnosis could be relevant to this comparison.

2 (a) The crude birth rate per thousand

$$= \frac{\text{number of births}}{\text{total population}} \times 1\,000$$

$$= \frac{68\,892}{5\,153\,300} \times 1\,000$$

$$= 13.4.$$

(b) The crude death rate per thousand

$$= \frac{\text{number of deaths}}{\text{total population}} \times 1\,000$$

$$= \frac{63\,299}{5\,153\,300} \times 1\,000$$

$$= 12.3.$$

(c) The general fertility rate per thousand

$$= \frac{\text{number of births}}{\text{number of women 15–44}} \times 1\,000$$

$$= \frac{68\,892}{1\,080\,600} \times 1\,000$$

$$= 63.8.$$

3 The doctor certifying the cause of death will enter stomach cancer as the cause on Mrs Wells' certificate of cause of death. This will go to the local registrar, and eventually to OPCS in London. Coders there will convert the information to an ICD number. Mrs Wells' death will then be added to the total of stomach cancer deaths for women of her age and last occupation, who lived in her part of the country. This total will be among the figures eventually published by OPCS.

Table 4.7 (answers)

District	Age group				
	0–19	20–39	40–64	65 and over	Total (= 100 %)
Milton Keynes	34.64	34.60	21.64	9.11	123 296
Aylesbury Vale	31.41	30.44	26.57	11.58	130 771

4 (a) The SMR is used because the age structure differs from one occupational group to another. If crude death rates were used, one group might appear to have a high death rate merely because it contained older men. Standardisation for age avoids this problem. Indirect standardisation was used here, giving SMRs. (Incidentally, the smoking figures were also age-standardised in much the same way as the death rates.)

(b) Taking the construction workers first, there were 44 per cent more deaths from lung cancer in this group than would have occurred had national age-specific death rates applied to the group. For sales workers, 15 per cent fewer deaths occurred than would have been the case if national rates had applied. Thus, allowing for age, lung cancer affects construction workers to a greater degree than sales workers.

5 First, the expectation of life at birth *in 1976* was 69.7, which is less than 45 + 27.8, as you saw on p. 42, because it is the mean lifetime of the whole of a cohort, whereas the 27.8 figure excludes those who died before the age of 45. Second, the expectation of life at birth in 1931 is less still, because age-specific death rates fell between 1931 and 1976. (Remember that life expectancy is the average length of life of a *hypothetical* cohort.)

6 (a) The incidence rate for 1982

$$= \frac{5}{56\,300} \times 100\,000$$

$$= 8.9 \text{ per } 100\,000.$$

(b) The prevalence rate at 30 June 1982

$$= \frac{119}{56\,300} \times 100\,000$$

$$= 211.4 \text{ per } 100\,000.$$

Chapter 6
1 (a) This was a retrospective case-control study, because it compared a group of cases with a group of controls, and looked back into their past history.

(b) No. With a case-control study, one finds a group of cases and a group of controls. It could then be worked out what proportion of people with lung cancer were heavy smokers, for example. But this is not the same thing as the proportion of heavy smokers who die from lung cancer. This can only be calculated by finding a group of smokers and *then* counting how many die of lung cancer, that is by doing a cohort study.

2 (a) Because there is no established cure, the other group may receive no active treatment. However, this control group should be given a placebo.

(b) At *random*.

(c) No, the doctor should not know, as this may bias the assessment in some way.

(d) 'The average rating of patients receiving the drug is the same as the average rating of those receiving the placebo.' (Note that the null hypothesis refers to the *average* ratings.)

(e) This does not *definitely* mean that the drug has no effect. It *may* have no effect; or it *may* be that the drug *does* have an effect, but the trial did not provide enough evidence to establish it.

Chapter 7
1 The simple answer is that social science is concerned with the *relationships* between individuals which shape their lives, not just with individuals. Epidemiology deals with large numbers of people but epidemiologists are primarily interested in the *distribution* of disease between individuals and not so interested in the nature of their relationships. (A more elaborate answer would say that although epidemiology examines groups of people, it does not deal with the social nature of those groups, the way they are formed by direct and indirect interactions and the manner in which those interactions both shape and are shaped by individual action — all of which have consequences for health.)

2 All three levels are referred to: the *individual* — 'Mr Lawson' and 'that doctor'; *direct interaction* — 'that doctor becomes anxious every time she sees Mr Lawson'; the *group* — 'doctor' refers to a group as well as to an individual. (Note that it is characteristic of speech to refer regularly to all three levels of social organisation.)

3 Direct interaction (with the chemist) is explicit. But the speaker is also linked, via a chain of indirect interaction, with all the people who package and distribute the tablets, or who own the company or the chemists. (If you thought really hard about this, you might have come up with a further instance of each type: the direct interaction of the speaker with whoever they were speaking to (we are not told), and the indirect interaction of the speaker with the reader and writers of this text.)

Chapter 8
1 (a) Observation would be used for (i), (ii) and (iii), experiment would be used for (iv) and (v) and animal modelling for (v).

(b) Accurate measurement should be possible in (iii) and (iv) but looks harder in (i), (ii) and (v).

(c) You might have thought of the following points. First, although chimps can help one another when ill (v), they do not perform hysterectomies or go to medical school! So we are forced to choose one or more of the other methods. Asking the surgeons (i) would obviously help, but even if they agree with our hypothesis, does it prove it? Filming their training (ii) sounds interesting and might tell us what it is about their training that produces variation in their criteria for hysterectomy — if our hypothesis is correct. But is it? Modifying the training selectively (iv), the experimental method, seems the best idea — but how do we persuade the medical schools to agree? And how long must we run the experiment before we can be sure of our results? Overall, the method that is both practical and reasonably effective would seem to be (iii), checking to see if there is any association between the surgeons' criteria and the medical schools they attended. Also, we should be able to measure that.

There is, however, one possible complication that might have struck you. What if our measurement showed no association? We could still not be sure that our hypothesis was wrong. Medical schools are large and complex, and change quite rapidly in some respects. Maybe there is an association, but only with particular teachers or student intakes. Interviewing the surgeons or filming their training might be less direct and harder to measure, but it might still have some real value after all. It would take us a lot further inside the medical school. Nor should we rule out experiment entirely. Even if we lack the power to alter the curriculum, we can still check to see if past changes in the curriculum or in the staffing or student intake are associated with our surgeons' varying criteria. In other words, instead of conducting our own experiments, we can look for 'natural experiments' and study their outcomes.

Chapter 9

1 (a) There are no 'ums', 'ers' or hesitations, and everything comes out in sentences. This is written, not spoken, speech. This suggests that it was either recorded by hand or, if a tape-recorder was used, that the transcriber has modified it to fit written conventions.

(b) Using 'observational' in the restricted sense found in social science, this latter speech is interview data. It consists of remarks made to the researcher by the doctor and is therefore different from his conversation with the mother, which is being observed and recorded by the researcher. (Note that off-the-cuff comments can sometimes be far more telling than those made in more formal interviews after the event.)

(c) The fact that the doctor said one thing to the mother and the social worker and another to the observer, suggests that observation can still uncover all kinds of backroom secrets. People do not necessarily alter their behaviour when observed. (However, maybe there is still some observer-effect. The doctor seems to be remarkably frank to the researcher. But, as you may have spotted, maybe this was because she was worried in case the observer had noticed the child's slight delay and felt obliged to justify herself.)

(d) There are several quantitative statements here — 'the end of January', and 'two or three months time' both refer to our system for counting time. You probably noticed those. But what about 'that was a difficult one' or 'I can't find any abnormalities'. These are still forms of quantification. To count one or none is still to count. This would have been more obvious if he'd gone on to remark, 'we've had two difficult cases today' or 'I can't find any abnormalities but there were three in that last case'.

(e) It tells us that official records are not always to be believed, even if they consist of statements by doctors to magistrates. (Qualitative researchers have conducted some fascinating studies of the rather murky processes by which official records and statistics are actually created.)

Chapter 10

1 (a) As the research is explicitly intended to facilitate the development of a large-scale service, the researchers would want numerical data in the main, and data that are relatively easy to analyse. They would therefore probably choose a structured interview survey.

(b) They would be most likely to choose face-to-face interviews (i) because elderly people might need more help than usual in filling in forms, and this might mean a postal survey (ii) would get a very low response. A telephone survey (iii) would similarly be inappropriate at least partly because the proportion of elderly people with a telephone is likely to be low. However, the face-to-face method is not without problems: for instance, the most vulnerable old people might be less likely to open their doors to a stranger.

2 Independence, like social class, is an aspect of the social world that is difficult to measure, and the researchers will have to find proxy measures.

There are many facets of independence and we have already touched on one possible dimension in the answer to question 1. The researchers could include proxy measures such as being able to clothe, cook and eat without help. They could also attempt to measure mobility, but asking about this could prove tricky. If the researchers ask the old people how easily they can get about, for instance, their answers may appear similar but mean very different things. More knowable or 'objective' measures, such as being able to get to the shops, to climb the stairs, or just to walk unaided, would allow the questions and answers to be more precise but do not tap the individual's subjective feelings about how independent they are. The researchers would probably use several different proxy measures, and the ones they choose will be largely determined by the research objectives.

Chapter 11

1 The word 'science' is being used in the following senses: (i) science as an *institution*; (ii) science as a *collection of methods*; (iii) science as a body of *facts* about the world.

2 (a) *Reductionist* Mr Lawson's genetic make-up resulted in a disordered biochemistry of his pancreatic cells: hence they could not produce insulin: hence his diabetes.

(b) *Holistic* Plumbing is a job that makes heavy physical demands on people, and the nature of the work and the pay associated with it, resulted in Mr Lawson adopting a diet that encouraged a genetic propensity to diabetes.

(c) *Temporal* Early childhood experience made Mr Lawson very prone to eating sweets and other foods containing carbohydrates. This resulted in him suffering diabetes.

3 The statements are: (a) fact; (b) theory; (c) fact; (d) theory.

4 (a) The government is acting on an essentially *functionalist* model. They are trying to set up a new system which they think will generate future harmony, even though it might create *conflict* in the present.

(b) Conflict theory.

(c) Opinions would differ. Some would see this in *functionalist* terms — a return to harmony. *Conflict theorists* would argue that the strikers were temporarily blinded by the ideology of the elite.

(d) Functionalist theory.

5 (a) Ethnicity.

(b) This is a genetic difference between a Jewish *population* and a population of non-Jewish people. Jews who do not originate from Eastern Europe do not show the same prevalence of disease, so this must mean that they are genetically different from the Eastern European Jews. Therefore Jews as a group cannot be regarded as a single race in the biological sense.

(c) This is an ethnic stereotype.

(d) This is a statement about the performance at school of different ethnic groups. It is thus a social statement. As the groups (Asian, Caribbean) do not form biologically defined races, there is no way that a biological explanation of this difference can be given.

Entries and page numbers in **bold type** refer to key words which are printed in *italics* in the text.

Index